A Nurse's Survival Guide to Supervising and Assessing

At Elsevier, we understand the importance of providing up-to-date and relevant content. For this reason, we are continuously working on updated editions and new titles for the Series. Please visit our website to find out the latest news and the upcoming publications : https://www.uk.elsevierhealth.com/

A Nurse's Survival Guide to Supervising and Assessing

Second Edition

Karen Elcock
Head of Programmes - Pre-Registration Nursing
Kingston University
Kingston upon Thames
United Kingdom

ELSEVIER

ISBN: 978-0-7020-8147-7

Content Strategist: Robert Edwards
Content Development Specialist: Andrae Akeh
Project Manager: Haritha Dharmarajan
Designer: Amy Buxton
Illustration Manager: Gopalakrishnan Venkatraman

Printed in India

Last digit is the print number: 9 8 7 6 5 4 3 2 1

Working together
to grow libraries in
developing countries

www.elsevier.com • www.bookaid.org

Contents

Chapter 1

Supporting Learning in Practice

Chapter Outline

INTRODUCTION

Practice placements are an essential part of pre-registration nursing programmes. It is an Nursing and Midwifery Council (NMC) requirement that student nurses spend 50% of their programmes learning in and from practice. However, learning in practice poses more challenges than learning at university. At university learning is scheduled with clearly set out timetables and confirmed dates for assessment that are set in stone. The delivery of theory is therefore predictable and enables students to plan theory learning. In practice, learning is less predictable. Whilst there are core elements that can be predicted as available as regular learning opportunities (e.g. medication rounds, observations), the constantly changing flow of patients and service users being cared for and sudden emergencies or unplanned changes in care means that learning in practice needs far more flexibility to enable students to learn. Alongside this is the need for sufficient staffing resources and the availability of appropriately prepared practice supervisors and assessors. This chapter looks at the importance of learning in practice, provides a brief overview of how roles for supporting learning in practice have developed over time and discusses the different influences leading to the changes by the NMC in their 2018 Standards and in how students

A Nurse's Survival Guide to Supervising and Assessing. https://doi.org/10.1016/B978-0-7020-8147-7.00001-6

are supported, supervised and assessed in practice. The final section provides an overview of some new models for supporting learning in practice currently being used in the UK.

THE IMPORTANCE OF LEARNING IN PRACTICE

It is unlikely that anyone would disagree that it is important that students learn the skills of nursing by participating in the real world of practice. The NMC *Code* (2018a) sets out its expectations of nurses, nursing associates and midwives with regard to their role in supporting and developing others, specifically stating that you are required to *'share your skills, knowledge and experience for the benefit of people receiving care and your colleagues and to support students' and colleagues' learning to help them develop their professional competence and confidence'*.

The opportunity to support and develop students and others can be incredibly gratifying. The benefits that can be gained from facilitating and developing the learning of others also provide intrinsic rewards that are unique within our profession. The prospect of being able to supervise, develop and make a lasting contribution to the learning needs of students is one to be valued as a key and fundamental aspect of your professional standing and career development.

To facilitate learning in practice student nurses have had supernumerary status since the 1980s, although interestingly students and staff in practice still frequently refer to this time in practice as working. Whilst students are expected to engage with and participate in the day-to-day activities that take place in practice, supernumerary status is a reminder that the student is additional to the workforce and this status is required to enable them to access the full opportunities for learning that are available. Exposure to learning opportunities and support from staff in practice is essential and provides a range of benefits that are important to develop well-rounded nurses.

Integration of Theory and Practice

In practice students learn how to apply and integrate the theory they learn at university to the real world of practice, with staff in practice playing a crucial role in enabling the student to make sense of this theory through participation in appropriate learning activities. The nature of nursing programmes and the challenges of placement capacity inevitably means that it is impossible for students to be taught all the theory relevant to a specific type of placement before they commence it. Some theory which is applicable to their placement will have been delivered before they start, some will be delivered later in the programme. This means that where students are involved in situations that they have not yet been taught about at university, they will need explanations and guidance on the theory supporting the practice seen or health conditions that are new to them. This new knowledge can then be used in future placements and also in university to support new theory learnt in future modules and the assessments they will be undertaking.

Professional Socialisation – Developing Their Identity as a Nurse

Whilst students are taught about the professional role of the nurse in university and prepared for practice through clinical skills and simulated learning, it is in practice that they fully develop their identity as a nurse. In practice they develop the behaviour, attitudes and values expected of the nursing profession. This is acquired by working alongside nurses learning how they deliver care, being exposed to expert practitioners and learning about the importance of teamwork including participation with the multidisciplinary team. However, students can find dissonance between what they are taught in university and what they see in practice. This encompasses not only the way skills may be delivered differently in practice but also in their expectations of how they will be supported to learn in practice and the reality when they get there.

While students have control over what they want to learn, they have limited control over access to the range of learning opportunities available to them. However, this can be achieved through discussion with their practice supervisors and assessor to identify what they wish to learn and what they need to learn so that access to the appropriate learning opportunities can be provided. Sadly, students report that 'Getting the work done' can become the mantra in practice especially at busy times, compromising their access to the learning opportunities they need, with students feeling like they are just an extra pair of hands (MacDonald et al., 2016). An alternative view for the practice supervisor to consider is 'how can the work that needs to be done today also enable a student to learn?' A lack of learning opportunities, feeling used to get the work done and lack of support from staff in practice will all impact on a student's satisfaction of their time on a placement and can impact on their decision to stay on their course.

Reducing Attrition in Pre-registration Nursing

Health Education England launched an investigation into student attrition in 2015 which culminated in the *RePAIR* report (Reducing Pre-registration Attrition and Improving Retention). One of the outcomes is an online toolkit available to universities and practice partners with examples of strategies to improve student retention during their programmes and in the first 2 years after starting employment. Although undertaken in England, it also includes information from organisations across the UK and so has applicability to all the devolved nations.

The report found that students' experiences of practice not only influenced their decision whether to leave or remain on their programme, particularly in the first year, but also influenced their decisions on which placement/organisation they decided to apply to on qualifying (Lovegrove, 2018). At that time mentors were seen by students as pivotal to the quality of the student experience and could make or break a placement for students, a view supported by many years of research into students' experiences in practice which have influenced the development of how students are supported in practice.

THE DEVELOPMENT OF ROLES TO SUPPORT STUDENT LEARNING IN PRACTICE

Mentorship was introduced by the former English National Board (ENB) for Nursing and Midwifery in the late 1980s. The term mentorship has always generated significant debate (Fulton, 2015) as the term 'mentor', which has its origins in Greek mythology, describes someone who is a guide or advisor to a younger or less experienced person. However, in nursing, whilst the initial guidance from the ENB was that the role was a supportive one and that the student should select their mentor, in reality students were allocated their mentor who was expected to not only support and supervise the student but also assess them (Fulton, 2015). The requirement to undertake this multiplicity of roles created conflict for mentors particularly when faced with a failing student. Kathleen Duffy's (2003) seminal work on failing students found that mentors saw failing a student as difficult. There were many reasons including feeling unsupported by lecturers from the university, the time involved and concerns on the impact on the student. Duffy's work influenced the NMC's development of new mentorship standards in 2006.

The NMC published their *Standards to Support Learning and Assessment in Practice* in 2006 and updated them in 2008 (NMC, 2008). During the time the NMC was consulting on the mentorship standards they were also consulting on fitness to practice at the point of registration. Both consultations highlighted concerns about the quality of the support students receive in practice and this along with Duffy's report, which had been published just before, led to a set of standards that were far more prescriptive than had been seen before with very specific requirements for the roles of mentors, practice teachers and teachers. The standards also introduced a new role of sign-off mentor, who had undertaken additional preparation and whose responsibility it was to confirm (sign off) students' proficiency in practice on their final placement (although all practice teachers and midwifery mentors had to be prepared as sign-off mentors). Each placement provider was required to keep a register of all mentors and sign-off mentors and ensure that they remained current (live) through annual updates and participation in a triennial review to demonstrate that they continued to meet the NMC's requirements set out in the standards. In addition, it was also an NMC requirement that "*Whilst giving direct care in the practice setting at least 40% of a student's time must be spent being supervised (directly or indirectly) by a mentor/practice teacher*" (NMC, 2008 p. 39).

The requirements of the *Standards for Learning and Assessment in Practice* (SLAiP) placed significant time and financial pressures on placement providers.

The cost in time and money in delivering the Standards was significant. Staff had to undertake NMC-approved mentorship programmes, attend annual updates and organisations had to maintain an accurate mentor register (in a profession which has a continual flow of staff across departments and between organisations). Whilst the SLAiP Standards allowed mentors to support up to three students, in reality most placement providers operated on one student per mentor, which required significant numbers of mentors to support the numbers of students placed with them. This approach to mentorship was highly problematic and did not resolve the problem of failing to fail.

Sir Robert Francis in his report into the events that took place at Mid Staffordshire Hospital (Francis, 2013) recommended that there was a need for the NMC to review their education standards. Around the same time a series of reports with a particular focus on nurse education were also published. Whilst the scope of each of them varied, they identified common themes related to the challenges of mentorship and practice learning. See Box 1.1 for a summary of four of the key reports that have influenced current models of student support in practice.

In 2016 the NMC commenced a major reform of both nursing and midwifery education including a new approach to the support of learning in practice. This resulted in the publication of a series of new standards for pre-registration nursing and nursing associate programmes, along with standards for return to practice programmes and nurse prescribers; standards for midwifery programmes were published in 2019. Separate but applicable to all of these programmes are the *Standards for student supervision and assessment* (NMC, 2018b). These last standards, commonly called the SSSA, introduced a significant change to the way that students would be supported. The changes reflect a response to the challenges discussed above, including:

- Replacing mentors with practice supervisors and practice assessors, thus separating the two roles which had long caused conflict.
- A defined role for lecturers (academic assessor) in the assessment process.
- A tripartite model with practice supervisors, practice assessors and academic assessors engaged in the student's learning journey in practice.

The new standards are explored in more detail in Chapter 2 but a key outcome was standards that were far more flexible than had been seen before and which would allow universities and their placement providers to consider more innovative approaches to programme delivery, including learning in practice.

MODELS OF LEARNING IN PRACTICE

The challenges in supporting learning in practice discussed earlier have seen the implementation of a number of new approaches to supporting learning in practice. Although the following models were initially designed prior to the introduction of the new NMC Standards in 2018, their approaches reflect many of the aims in the new standards.

BOX 1.1 Summary of key reports related to mentorship and practice learning

Quality with compassion: The future of nursing education Report of the Willis Commission on Nursing Education, 2012.	• Need to enhance the quality of many practice learning experiences. • Managers, mentors, practice education facilitators and academic staff must work together to help students relate theory to practice. • Dedicated time needed for mentors who are supported and valued.
Raising the bar shape of caring: A review of the Future Education and Training of Registered Nurses and Care Assistants, 2015 by Lord Willis	• More advanced skills needed, including diagnostic, prescribing and clinical and communication skills. • Review current mentorship modules and consider alternatives to 1:1 mentorship such as the Collaborative Learning in Practice model. • Introduce an annual nursing undergraduate survey. • Standardised assessments recommended.
Evaluation of the NMC pre-registration standards: Summary report, 2015 by IFF Research.	• National Health Service (NHS) Trusts and Health Boards to discourage rules which limit students' opportunities to practise essential skills. • Standardised Practice Assessment Booklets across universities. • Closer relationships and information sharing between practice and universities. • Consider whether mentor and sign-off mentor roles should be distinct or combined. • Review sustainability of the 1:1 mentorship model. • Prepare students to become mentors as part of the curriculum.
RCN Mentorship Project 2015 (Bazian Ltd., 2016)	• Change from 1:1 mentoring model to more peer-/team-based mentoring models for example. • Real Life Learning Wards, for example Collaborative Learning in Practice model. • Dedicated Education Units. • Clinical Facilitation Models.

Collaborative Learning in Practice

The Collaborative Learning in Practice (CLiP) model originated in Amsterdam and was introduced into the UK in 2014; it has been shown to have a number of benefits for students (Hill et al., 2020). It has been adopted and adapted by an increasing number of universities across the UK in collaboration with their placement providers as it offers an approach to increase placement capacity (Bazian Ltd, 2016). It has primarily been implemented in adult and community nursing settings but Hirdle and Keeley (2020) have evaluated its use in child and adolescent mental health services. CLiP uses a coaching model with a registered nurse acting as a coach to a small group of students who are assigned a group of patients for whom they plan and deliver care. Students delegate care, liaise with multidisciplinary teams and lead on the decision-making process. This approach also enables peer learning and the development of leadership skills for senior students as they work alongside their peers. Box 1.2 lists the roles and responsibilities for each person involved in the CLiP process.

BOX 1.2 Roles involved in Collaborative Learning in Practice

Roles involved in CLiP	Responsibilities
Student	Allocated maximum of three patients
	Identifies own learning needs
	Supports other students
	Predominantly the caregivers
Coach	Registered professional who works in the service
	Provides supervision and coaching during shift
	Responsible for care provided and quality of learning experiences
	No other roles during shift
Practice educator	Supports coaches and staff in practice
	Provides resources and guidance
	Works with teams to maximise learning opportunity
Coaching team	Students have opportunity to work with other staff in team
	All staff are responsible for ensuring quality of learning environment
Assessor	Registered nurse
	Reviews student learning
	Responsible for final assessment
	Gains feedback and evidence from other team members on students' performance
University	Provides training and support for coaches in practice
	Conduit between university and practice
	Lead for adherence to standards and quality

(Adapted from Hirdle and Keeley, 2020.)

BOX 1.3 Comparison of mentorship with the Collaborative Learning in Practice model

Traditional mentorship in nursing	The CLiP model
Must be a registered nurse	Any registered health and social care practitioner
1:1 model	
Directs learning	1: many model
Mentor acts as supervisor and teacher, tells what and how	Students take responsibility for their learning
	Coach uses questions and guides students to seek answers
Longer-term relationship	
Student focusses on mentor	Short-term relationship
	Students learn with and from peers
	Develops leadership skills in senior students

CLiP, Collaborative Learning in Practice.
(Adapted from Hill et al., 2020.)

As you can see the CLiP model aligns well with the new SSSA Standards with a practice supervisor coaching the student group across the length of a shift and practice assessors meeting with their student(s) at key points during their placement to evaluate their learning, identify areas for further learning and ensure the students are on target for on-time completion of their practice assessment documents. For practice supervisors there is however a fundamental change in the way they support students using CLiP, which is very different from previous mentoring approaches which are summarised in Box 1.3. Key is the focus on coaching skills which use questioning skills to enable students to find the answers themselves rather than telling students the answers and what they need to do.

The Strengthening Team-based Education in Practice model

The Strengthening Team-based Education in Practice (STEP) model was a project led by Middlesex University in collaboration with colleagues from a number of universities in London and their practice partners. The model recognises that learning in practice requires a team-based approach involving a range of people who can support student learning. The project resulted in some web-based resources and a publication (Morley et al., 2019). The approach is based on five themes that can assist practitioners to plan for and develop their role in supporting pre-registration nursing students. These themes are:

- Comprehensive orientation and socialisation – emphasises the importance of orientation to the placement, with students being welcomed and enabled to feel they belong as part of the nursing and healthcare team.
- The role of 'Helpful Others' – explores the role of healthcare assistants and others not normally considered as having a role to play in supporting student learning in practice, including other members of the multidisciplinary team.

- Student peer support/learning – emphasises the value of peer support and learning with and from peers in practice.
- Academic-practice partnership work – in-line with the new NMC SSSA standards this area focusses on the development of partnership working between practice and the university.
- Expansive learning – explores a coaching model that can be used to develop students through their learning journey in practice.

Resources to support the implementation of STEP are available on-line and the link can be found at the end of this chapter.

Learning in practice is highly valued by students and their experiences in practice will shape the registered nurse they will become. Your role as a practice supervisor or practice assessor is pivotal, therefore, in shaping the future workforce and in encouraging recruitment to your area of work. The chapters which follow in this book will provide you with strategies to plan for students allocated to your placement and explore strategies to support them to enable a positive experience for you and for them.

NURSING ASSOCIATE STUDENTS AND STUDENT NURSE/ NURSING ASSOCIATE APPRENTICESHIPS

The principles within this chapter apply equally to students on nursing apprenticeship programmes and apprentice student nurses/nursing associates. The key difference will be with apprenticeship students who will have periods in practice when they are supernumerary across a range of settings to meet NMC requirements and periods when they are undertaking work-based learning within their base placement. Nursing associate apprentices will require protected time within their base placement and the hours required for this will be provided by the student's university.

Action points

- Review the Royal College of Nursing (RCN) *Practice-based learning* website (see below for links) and consider whether any of the models described could be implemented in your own workplace.
- Discuss some of the ideas you have seen on the RCN website and in this chapter with colleagues at work to gauge interest in trialling something new.
- Talk to the lead for education in your organisation about ideas you would like to try out and ask for their support.

USEFUL WEBSITES

RCN Practice-based learning available at: https://www.rcn.org.uk/professional-development/practice-based-learning

STEP (Strengthening Team-based Education in Practice) available at: https://www.stepapproach-learning.org/

Chapter 2

NMC Standards for Pre-registration Nursing

Chapter Outline

INTRODUCTION

In order to support student learning in practice it is essential to have an understanding of the NMC standards underpinning the programme they are undertaking. The standards set out what is required of universities, academic staff, practice learning partners and all health and social care professionals who support students in practice. Within each of their standards related to educational programmes for nurses, midwives nursing associates and students on return to practice programmes, the NMC sets out a number of requirements, which are prefaced by the statement: *Approved education institutions, together with practice learning partners, must….* In making this statement the NMC is clearly articulating the requirement for partnership working and an equal responsibility for the delivery of the programmes these standards relate to. The standards related to pre-registration nursing will have been used to develop the curriculum for the nursing programmes run by your local universities with regard to both their structure and content and therefore an understanding of what is expected of both universities and staff in practice is important if these standards are to be met. This chapter summarises the four standards that underpin pre-registration nursing programmes and why they are important for practice supervisors and assessors supporting students in practice.

THE NURSING AND MIDWIFERY COUNCIL STANDARDS

In 2018 the NMC published a series of new standards which required universities to revalidate their programmes in partnership with practice partners and to rethink their approach for learning in practice. The new standards were developed for pre-registration nursing, nursing associate and post-registration programmes (return to practice and nurse prescribing), with new standards for midwifery programmes published in 2019.

At the time of writing the NMC is still reviewing their post-registration standards for specialist community public health nursing (SCPHN) and specialist practice qualifications (SPQ). All universities were required to move to the new standards for nursing, nursing associates and return to practice and nursing and midwifery prescribers by September 2020, and to the new standards for pre-registration midwifery programmes by September 2021.

The NMC's Realising Professionalism: Standards for Education and Training are set out in three parts:

Part 1: Standards framework for nursing and midwifery education
Part 2: Standards for student supervision and assessment
Part 3: Programme standards:
- Standards for pre-registration nursing programmes
- Standards for pre-registration midwifery programmes
- Standards for pre-registration nursing associate programmes
- Standards for return to practice programmes
- Standards for prescriber programmes

At the same time as publishing the new standards the NMC removed their 2007 Standards for medicines management because as a regulator it was not appropriate for them to provide clinical practice guidelines. The NMC website does however provide links to key standards related to medicines management available from Health Education England, the Royal Pharmaceutical Society and the Royal College of Nursing that nurses and midwives can access for guidance.

The standards listed above not only set out the requirements of the NMC but also include (for pre-registration nursing and midwifery programmes) the requirements set out in the EU Directive on the *recognition of professional qualifications* (Directive 2005/36/EC of the European Parliament, amended by Directive 2013/55/EU). The Directive sets out the broad requirements for nursing and midwifery programmes including the length of the programmes, recognition of prior learning (RPL), hours of theory and practice required in each programme, the use of simulation and key areas of content which must be included in these programmes. Whilst the Directives for nursing relate to adult nursing only, the NMC requires all fields to meet the directives in relation to RPL, length of programmes and hours of theory and practice that must be met. The relevant sections of the EU Directive on nursing are provided by the NMC in Annexe 1 of Part 3 of the NMC's *Standards for pre-registration nursing programmes* (NMC, 2018c). The EU Directive ensures a shared recognition of a number of health professional qualifications enabling free flow of healthcare professionals across the European Union and the UK on the basis that programmes meet a common standard. The Directives also include requirements for language checks and a duty for each country to share information regarding banned or suspended healthcare professionals (Royal College of Nursing, 2019). Nursing, nursing associate and midwifery programmes each have their own separate standards of proficiency reflecting their different roles and responsibilities.

The key areas covered in each of the Standards related to nursing are summarised in Box 2.1. Each standard is only a few pages in length and should be read by anyone involved in the education of students. They are available to read online or download from the NMC website: www.nmc.org.uk/standards.

THE STANDARDS FOR STUDENT SUPERVISION AND ASSESSMENT

These standards, commonly called the SSSA, apply to all NMC-approved programmes and set out the NMC's expectations for the learning, support and supervision of students within practice learning environments and their assessment in theory and practice. The SSSA replaced the previous NMC *Standards for learning and assessment in practice* (SLAiP) (NMC, 2008), which applied to mentors, practice teachers and teachers. One of the aims of the new standards was to provide both universities and practice partners the opportunity for greater flexibility and creativity in how they develop and implement practice learning experiences for students. In addition, they addressed some of the concerns related to the SLAiP standards discussed in Chapter 1, which are summarised in Box 2.2.

BOX 2.1 Summary of NMC 2018 Future Nurse Standards

NMC standard	Key sections
Part 1: Standards framework for nursing and midwifery education	1. Learning culture 2. Educational governance and quality 3. Student empowerment 4. Educators and assessors 5. Curricula and assessment

Part 2: Standards for student supervision and assessment	Effective practice learning
	  1. Organisation of practice learning
	Supervision of students
	  2. Expectations of practice supervision
	  3. Practice supervisors: role and responsibilities
	  4. Practice supervisors: contribution to assessment and progression
	  5. Practice supervisors: preparation
	Assessment of students and confirmation of proficiency
	  6. Assessor roles
	  7. Practice assessors: responsibilities
	  8. Practice assessors: preparation
	  9. Academic assessors: responsibilities
	  10. Academic assessors: preparation

Part 3: Standards for pre-registration nursing programmes	1. Selection, admission and progression 2. Curriculum 3. Practice learning 4. Supervision and assessment 5. Qualification to be awarded
Future nurse: Standards of proficiency for registered nurses	Platform 1: Being an accountable professional Platform 2: Promoting health and preventing ill health Platform 3: Assessing needs and planning care Platform 4: Providing and evaluating care Platform 5: Leading and managing nursing care and working in teams Platform 6: Improving safety and quality of care Platform 7: Coordinating care Annexe A: Communication and relationship management skills Annexe B: Nursing procedures

BOX 2.2 Changes to Supervision/Assessor Roles Following Implementation of the SSSA

Requirements in the SLAiP Standards (2008)	Changes with the SSSA
All mentors to complete an NMC-approved mentorship programme	Preparation programmes no longer need to be approved by the NMC
A register of mentors to be maintained and updated	No register required although most organisations are keeping a record of assessors and supervisors
Annual updates and triennial reviews	No formal requirement but all registrants undertake revalidation every 3 years and should demonstrate that they maintain their competence as a practice supervisor/assessor
Due regard for field of practice	Practice assessors (and academic assessors) must be registered nurses with appropriate equivalent experience for a student's field of practice

SLAiP, Standards for learning and assessment in practice; SSSA, standards for student supervision and assessment.

Whilst due regard for field of practice is no longer required, both practice assessors and academic assessors supporting student nurses must be registered nurses (or registered nurses/nursing associates to support student nursing associates). Although the NMC no longer requires practice partners to maintain a register of staff involved in supervising and assessing students, it does expect placement providers and universities to be assured that there are sufficient practice supervisors/assessors to support students in practice. Most organisations have decided to maintain a register of assessors and supervisors as this information is required so that they know how many practice supervisors/assessors they have in each placement and so how many students can be allocated to each area. It also enables them to know whether further preparation is needed to develop staff into these roles to ensure sufficient numbers to support current and future student numbers. Universities will also hold a record of academic staff who have been prepared to become academic assessors.

The SSSA sets out the NMC's expectations for the learning, support and supervision of students in the practice environment. They also set out how students are assessed for theory and practice (NMC, 2018b). The standards apply to all NMC-approved programmes and are applicable to all settings where students learn. This means that even areas that just take students for a day or so as an outreach or spoke placement should be aware of them as they will be supervising students who spend time with them and so need to be aware of their learning needs. It is important therefore that there is effective communication from the student's main placement on what they will be aiming to achieve on an outreach placement and if the student has any additional support needs that need to be taken into account.

! The NMC have developed a website called **Supporting information on standards for student supervision and assessment** (the SISSA website) which provides a series of guides to help you understand and implement the SSSA, which are available here:

https://www.nmc.org.uk/supporting-information-on-standards-for-student-supervision-and-assessment/

The SSSSA standards are set out under three headings and are summarised by the NMC (2018b, p. 4) as follows:

- **Effective practice learning:** what needs to be in place to deliver safe and effective learning experiences for nursing and midwifery students in practice.
- **Supervision of students:** the principles of student supervision in the practice environment, and the role of the practice supervisor.
- **Assessment of students and confirmation of proficiency:** the role and responsibilities of the practice assessor and the academic assessor and what is required from each of these roles in assessing and confirming students' practice and academic achievement.

The academic assessor was a new role introduced in the SSSA standards that supports the student's journey through both theory and practice. This role complements that of the practice assessor but with a focus on the learning within the academic environment as opposed to learning in practice.

In reading the standards you will notice that the NMC has clearly demarcated responsibilities between the two very separate activities of supervising and assessing. This was warmly received by many academics and practitioners who had long argued that the role of assessor is incongruent with the previous role of a mentor, who is defined as someone who acts as a guide, friend and counsellor. The role of mentor had caused confusion and conflict for staff that had to switch between supporting and supervising students in practice to then making assessment decisions regarding a student's competence in practice. Let's look at *effective practice learning* and *supervision of students* in more detail and then explore the three roles of practice supervisor, practice assessor and academic assessor further.

Effective Practice Learning

To ensure that a practice placement is an effective learning environment for students, the university and practice partners need to demonstrate partnership working. For example, universities will have worked in partnership with their placement providers to develop their curriculum against the NMC standards and agreed on an approach to the implementation of the SSSA. In many cases partnership working extends across universities and placement providers. For example, in London the *Pan London Practice Learning Group* developed a Pan London Practice Assessment Document (PLPAD) and a pan London approach to implementing the SSSA across multiple universities and placement providers. This collaborative approach has included the development of a website with resources for all Higher Education Institutes (HEIs) and practice partners across the London area to access and aid them in implementing the standards. Similar approaches have been used across other regions in England who have adapted the PLPAD for their own use. In addition, Wales has a *'Once for Wales 2020'* strategy, Scotland a *'Once for Scotland'* strategy and Northern Ireland a *Future Nurse Future Midwife NMC Education Standards Northern Ireland (NI) Implementation* strategy. These pan region/country approaches have meant that placement providers who support students from more than one university no longer have to deal with different practice assessment documents. It also has led to common approaches to preparing staff in practice for their roles in supporting students. This is a significant benefit for placement providers and registered nurses as movement from one organisation to another is less likely to require significant updating of staff when they move to new organisations.

Governance and Educational Audits

Governance of practice learning is also essential to ensure that practice placements meet NMC requirements set out in their standards. This is managed in a number of ways including through educational audits of practice placements to ensure that the learning environment is suitable for students. The NMC does not specify what type of tool is used to audit the quality of a learning environment but does set out its expectations in their *Standards framework for nursing and midwifery education* (NMC, 2018e). To meet the NMC's requirements the following are key questions that may be asked as part of an educational audit:

- Are there sufficient numbers of appropriately prepared practice supervisors and practice assessors for the type and number of students that will be allocated to that area?
- Does the placement demonstrate a learning culture that reflects the values of the *Code* (NMC, 2018a)?
- Are appropriate policies and procedures in place including incidents and accidents?
- Are risk assessments in place that are kept under review?
- Is there a nominated person for each placement who can support students and address their concerns (e.g. a Practice Educator, the lead for placements/education in the organisation)?

Roles and responsibilities of practice supervisors and assessors must be clearly articulated and understood (definitions of the roles and responsibilities for key roles may be detailed in the practice assessment document and in student handbooks and guides for practice supervisors and assessors).

Both the university and placement providers need to ensure that the equality and diversity needs of students are taken into account. This will include making reasonable adjustments for students with a disability (see Chapter 10) as well as meeting other needs that recognise the diversity of students such as enabling religious needs, for example a modified uniform or flexible shift arrangements related to holy days.

Supervision of Students

All students must be supervised when they are in practice, but the level of supervision will depend on their individual learning needs. Unlike the former SLAiP standards which required students to be supervised (directly or indirectly) for 40% of their time in practice, the SSSA are less specific, advising that the level of supervision provided will depend on the needs of each individual student. First-year students would normally require more supervision than a final-year student. However, a final-year student may require close supervision when undertaking new skills, for example if practising cannulation for the first time, but as their confidence and competence grows then less supervision would be required. This ensures that the level of supervision can be tailored to each student's needs and may increase or decrease depending on their proficiency in different areas of practice or as they are required to learn new skills.

PRACTICE SUPERVISORS

The NMC *Code* (2018a) makes clear that it is your responsibility as a registered nurse, midwife or nursing associate to contribute to practice learning; this will include acting as a practice supervisor to students on NMC-approved programmes. Practice supervisors are seen as role models who demonstrate safe and effective practice to students. The NMC also allows other health and social care professionals who are registered with a professional regulator (e.g. midwives, nursing associates, doctors, physiotherapists, occupational therapists, paramedics, dieticians, pharmacists, social workers, etc.) to also act as practice supervisors. This provides greater flexibility in who might support and supervise students in practice and opens up a wider range of learning environments that are available to students to learn in, thus potentially expanding placement capacity. Students can be allocated to more than one practice supervisor, but it is essential that there is clarity on a day-to-day basis as to who is supervising the student, otherwise the student can be left in limbo unsure who is supervising them and who to go to if they have questions. Allocation of named practice supervisors therefore is essential and will need to be recorded in the practice assessment document.

! A practice supervisor cannot also be a practice assessor to the same student (and vice versa).

Role of the Practice Supervisor

The expectations of the practice supervisor are that they will act as a role model for students and support, supervise and provide them with feedback on their progress in achieving their proficiencies/learning outcomes. The named practice supervisor will generally be responsible for the induction to a placement and the initial interview and identifying the learning opportunities for the student to achieve their proficiencies.

! Check with your local university or read the practice assessment document on the roles and responsibilities for practice supervisors/assessors. Universities will have agreed with practice partners what sections of a practice assessment document can be completed and/or assessed by the practice assessor and practice supervisors.

The practice supervisor will record their observations of the student's progress in the practice assessment document and may, if agreed by the university and their practice partners, also sign off achievement of professional values (most likely at mid-point only) and learning outcomes/proficiencies as long as they are within their scope of practice. For example, an adult nurse may be supervised by a psychiatric liaison nurse during an accident and emergency placement to enable them to learn about the assessment and support of people with suicidal ideation, or a learning disabilities student may spend time with a physiotherapist to learn techniques for postural care for people with profound and multiple disabilities. In both cases the practice supervisor would be expected to provide feedback to the practice assessor on the student's achievement of meeting the learning outcomes/proficiencies relevant to that experience, either directly or through documentation in the practice assessment document. The provision of feedback on a student's learning and achievement is an important part of the role of the practice supervisor as well as providing feedback on any areas of concerns regarding the student's conduct or competence.

Preparation of Practice Supervisors

The method for preparing practice supervisors is a decision between universities and their practice partners and may include face-to-face workshops or the use of on-line modules. The NMC no longer stipulates an approved course is required for preparing those who support student learning in practice. It does however state the minimum expectations of a practice supervisor, which are to:

- Understand the programme and proficiencies that students need to achieve.
- Be supported to develop skills to support student learning such as identifying learning opportunities, setting objectives, supervision and coaching skills, questioning skills, providing feedback and using reflection with students.

Role of Other Health and Social Care Professionals in Supporting and Supervising Students

As already discussed, the SSSA permits other registered health and social care professionals to supervise students. In most professions there are preparation programmes to prepare health and social care professionals to supervise and assess students from their own field of practice. This means they are likely to have an appropriate skill set in supervising and supporting students in practice. However, they will need preparation to understand the nursing student's programme and the proficiencies they need to achieve. This may be undertaken through short workshops, access to generic on-line preparation programmes for practice supervisors and the use of handbooks and guides from the university.

Health and social care practitioners provide students with access to a wider range of learning opportunities and enable them to practise skills that a nursing practice assessor may not have experience of. For example, dieticians are highly skilled in behaviour change, motivational interviewing and mindfulness, skills all four fields need to demonstrate to meet the NMC's proficiencies. Other non-registered health and social care professional such as phlebotomists, teachers, associate practitioners and healthcare assistants may also be able to contribute to a student's learning but cannot be practice assessors. We will consider this further in Chapter 6.

ASSESSMENT OF STUDENTS AND CONFIRMATION OF PROFICIENCY

As the standards are flexible and less prescriptive than prior standards each university and practice partnership may use a different approach towards the assessment and confirmation of students so if you move to a new organisation you may find some differences in how they have implemented the SSSA and what is required from you. As identified earlier there are two assessor roles: practice assessors and academic assessors. Practice assessors make decisions regarding the student's achievement in practice. Academic assessors check and confirm the student's achievement of their proficiencies and their programme requirements at university and confirm they can progress to the next part of the programme.

! A part of a programme is defined by the university and practice partners and approved at the point of validation. It relates to the point when a student progresses from one part of the programme to the next, for pre-registration nursing and nursing associates this is likely to be the end of each academic year.

For pre-registration nursing students the practice assessor and academic assessor must be registered nurses and have relevant and comparable experience for that student's field of practice. The experience could be either from their roles in practice or through completion of a recognised course relevant to a field of practice. For example, a health visitor may be a registered adult nurse but works with children and families so will have the appropriate work-based experience in order to assess child field students in practice or a lecturer who was a health visitor could be an academic assessor to a child field student at the university. A school nurse could be a registered adult nurse but works with children with special needs so could be a practice assessor to child field or learning disability students. Equally a learning disability nurse working with service users who are experiencing mental health problems will have the relevant work-based experience to act as a practice assessor to both learning disability and mental health students. For nursing associate students their practice assessor and academic assessor can be a registered nurse or a registered nursing associate.

Practice Assessors

Each student is nominated a practice assessor either for a single placement, across one or more placements, or for the whole part of the programme. The first option is likely to be the most common approach. It is the practice assessor who signs off a student's proficiency for a placement or for several placements across one part of a programme.

The option for a practice assessor to assess a student across more than one placement offers universities and placement providers the ability to utilise placements where there may not be staff who can be a practice assessor or there is only one staff member who is the practice supervisor so cannot be a practice assessor as well. For example, a student is allocated a practice assessor on a hospital ward and is then allocated to a General Practice (GP) surgery with only one registered nurse available who acts as their practice supervisor. In this situation the student would need a nominated practice assessor from another organisation to sign off their proficiencies achieved in the GP surgery; this could be their practice assessor from their previous placement. Whilst a student can have the same practice assessor across one or more placements, they cannot have the same practice assessor for two consecutive parts of a programme.

Role of the Practice Assessor

Practice assessors are responsible for signing off a student's achievement of their proficiencies and programme outcomes in practice for the period they are assigned to them, be it a placement or series of placements. At a progression point (end of a part) the practice assessor will also make recommendations for progression in collaboration with the academic assessor (this may be through a meeting, a telephone call or through documentation in the practice assessment document). Practice assessors must ensure they have a sound understanding of the student's programme and the proficiencies to be achieved. All decisions must be based on evidence; this means that they use a range of evidence to make their decision, including:

- Information recorded in the student's practice assessment document
- Feedback from the practice supervisor(s)
- Observation of the student in practice
- Discussions and reflection with the student.

In addition, the assessment must be objective and fair, which means that the practice assessor must take into account any reasonable adjustments the student requires (see Chapter 10). Fairness also means that where a student is not making the progress expected they should be provided with feedback and support in order to have the opportunity to improve and all decisions must be clearly documented. We will explore the assessment process and confirmation of proficiencies in Chapter 9.

Preparation of Practice Assessors

For staff who have completed a previously recognised mentorship programme, it is likely that placement providers have chosen to automatically transfer them over to the role of practice assessor with updating of the new standards and the programmes the students are undertaking. For staff who have not previously been a mentor they will need to undertake a preparation programme. The format of the programme will have been agreed between the university and the practice partners. The programme could be delivered as a workshop or on-line but the NMC (2018c, p. 10) identifies the following content as a minimum:

- Interpersonal communication skills, relevant to student learning and assessment
- Conducting objective, evidence-based assessments of students
- Providing constructive feedback to facilitate professional development in others
- Knowledge of the assessment process and their role within it.

Transitioning From Mentor/Sign-Off Mentor to Practice Supervisor/Practice Assessor

All practitioners who have an NMC-approved mentorship/practice teacher qualification and have continued to undertake this role should feel comfortable with the role of both practice supervisor and assessor as your programme will have prepared you for both supervising and assessing students. The difference now is that these two roles have been separated to enable a more robust approach to assessment. Change can be challenging but reflection on the expectations of the new roles should enable you to realise that you have the skills required but you will need to be updated on the responsibilities of the new roles. You will also need an understanding of the curriculum the students are undertaking and proficiencies they need to achieve.

> ! Read *A National Framework for Practice Supervisors, Practice Assessors and Academic Assessors in Scotland* (NHS Education for Scotland, 2019) which includes a mapping document for mentors/sign-off mentors and practice teachers to undertake a reflective self-assessment against the NMC practice supervisor and practice assessor roles.

Academic Assessors

Academic assessors were introduced as a new role in the SSSA standards to strengthen protection of the public by ensuring students are fit to practise (i.e. of good health and good conduct) at the point of registration. They are usually a member of the academic team delivering the programme at the university.

Role of the Academic Assessor

The academic assessor will review the student's progress through a part of the programme and ensure that they have achieved the proficiencies and programme outcomes in the academic environment in order to progress to the next part of the programme or on to registration if at the end of the programme. In addition, they will check there are no concerns regarding the student's conduct. They draw on a wide range of evidence including from practice and other sources (e.g. progress in previous parts, personal tutor, etc.)

Preparation of Academic Assessors

Academic assessors will either hold a relevant teaching qualification as required by their university or be working towards completion of it. The NMC defines the minimum outcomes an academic assessor must demonstrate as:

- Interpersonal communication skills, relevant to student learning and assessment
- Conducting objective, evidence-based assessments of students
- Providing constructive feedback to facilitate professional development in others
- Knowledge of the assessment process and their role within it (NMC, 2018b, p. 11)

FIG. 2.1 **Supervisor and assessor relationships.**

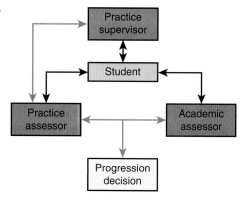

Clearly, they also need to have an understanding of the student's programme and must continue to develop themselves professionally and be supported to reflect on this role (this can be through annual appraisal and the NMC revalidation process each year).

The Relationship Between the Practice Assessor and Academic Assessor

The academic assessor works in partnership with the practice assessor to evaluate the student's achievement of the course requirements (theory and practice) and recommend the student for progression at the end of each part of the programme (Fig. 2.1). The NMC require the academic assessor and the practice assessor to communicate regarding a student's progress but do not define how this communication takes place. This will have been agreed locally between the university and their practice partners and could include scheduled meetings (face to face, by phone, email or on-line) and/or through recording their observations of the student's performance and areas for improvement within the Practice Assessment Document and Ongoing Achievement Record. Where a student is progressing well in practice less communication is likely to be required but where there are concerns that the student is not making the progress expected or there are concerns regarding their health or conduct then more frequent communication between the two assessors will be required. We will look at this in more detail in Chapter 8.

MAINTAINING YOUR COMPETENCE AS A PRACTICE ASSESSOR OR PRACTICE SUPERVISOR

Once you are confirmed as a practice supervisor or assessor that is not the end! You should receive support to continue to develop your role. This will come in part through your experience in supervising and assessing students but also through revalidation and reflecting on those experiences. Whilst the NMC does not specifically require you to update annually and no longer require a triennial review of your role as a supervisor/assessor, they do expect you to actively engage in activities to develop your role. This may include:

- Attending updates on the programmes you support and assess students on, provided by the universities who place students with you (this could be face to face, on-line or accessing materials from a website provided by the university)
- A discussion group with colleagues exploring successes and challenges you have encountered supporting students and how they were managed
- Study days related to coaching, supervision and assessment or that develop skills useful to your role (e.g. use of reflection, managing conflict, equality and diversity updates)
- Reading books or articles related to student support and assessment in practice. A number of nursing journals regularly publish articles relevant to supporting and assessing students and often these will have a series of activities for you to undertake while reading through them
- Developing materials to support student learning in your placement
- Attending seminars and conferences that focus on practice education
- Joining a professional group that focusses on practice education, for example the Royal College of Nursing (RCN) Education Forum
- Participating or leading on educational audits of practice placements in your organisation
- Participating in curriculum development groups at your local university
- Participation in OSCEs/OSCAs (objective structured clinical examinations/ assessments) or skills and simulation at your local university. This method of updating also provides an opportunity to discuss assessment of practice learning and in particular the challenges of ensuring the reliability and validity of assessments.

Whichever methods you use, ensure to remain up to date; remember to record them in your revalidation portfolio with the dates and type of activities undertaken, together with any additional evidence you may have of updating and feedback from students on your role in supervising or assessing them, as you will need this for your 3-yearly revalidation with the NMC.

FUTURE NURSE: STANDARDS OF PROFICIENCY FOR REGISTERED NURSES

The standards of proficiency set out the *knowledge and skills that registered nurses must demonstrate when caring for people of all ages and across all care settings* (NMC, 2018d, p. 3). They were developed to prepare students for their role as autonomous practitioners in a rapidly changing healthcare environment. They will ensure nurses in the future are equipped with the range of skills needed to care for people across the lifespan and across a range of healthcare environments. The proficiencies apply to all four fields of practice and are divided into seven platforms and two annexes. The platforms are:

1. Being an accountable professional
2. Promoting health and preventing ill health
3. Assessing needs and planning care
4. Providing and evaluating care
5. Leading and managing nursing care and working in teams
6. Improving safety and quality of care
7. Coordinating care

Each platform has a number of outcome statements which students have to achieve by the end of their programme; much of this will be achieved through the academic programme at university but some will be achieved in practice. The annexes set out the skills that each student must also be able to demonstrate by the end of their programme. Annexe A details the communication and relationship management skills and Annexe B provides a list of the nursing procedures students are required to develop proficiency in.

The skills annexes have created a lot of discussion and debate between universities and practice partners. The NMC expects that the student will be assessed on each of these skills within their own field of practice; however some of the skills pose a challenge for some fields of practice. The NMC recognises this, so whilst the proficiency outcomes and skills must be achieved by students from all four fields of practice, they note that the level of expertise that the student will demonstrate in some of the skills will vary depending on their field of practice but should be at a level appropriate to that field of practice. For example, a child or adult field student is likely to develop a greater level of expertise in chest auscultation than a mental health student. Conversely, a learning disability or mental health student will develop a greater level of proficiency in recognising and responding to challenging behaviour and in providing the appropriate safe holding and restraint if required. Familiarity with the practice assessment document used by your local universities will help you to identify which of the skills and proficiencies in the document are ones that students can achieve in your placement area and which ones may pose more of a challenge for students to gain learning opportunities in, in order to achieve them.

Prescribing

You will also notice when reading through the *Standards of Proficiency* that there is a greater emphasis on skills and knowledge related to prescribing. All students will be prepared through both their academic programme and experience in practice to be ready at the point of registration to go on to undertake a prescribing course. A newly qualified nurse could undertake an approved NMC prescribing programme which enables them to prescribe from the limited community formulary (NMC, 2018d). However, it should be noted that to undertake the supplementary/independent prescribing programme, a nurse or midwife must have been registered with the NMC for a minimum of 1 year before they can commence the V300 programme.

Getting to grips with the NMC's Standards can be difficult. Attendance at workshops to prepare you for the role of practice assessor or practice supervisor as well as workshops run by your local universities to update you on their programmes are all valuable ways to enable you to become more familiar with them. Many universities also provide on-line resources that are helpful in aiding you to understand the local context and are worth exploring.

THE NMC STANDARDS FOR NURSING DEGREE APPRENTICES AND NURSING ASSOCIATES

All of the NMC pre-registration nursing standards discussed apply equally to Registered Nurse Degree Apprentices (RDNA) as they do for UCAS (Universities and Colleges Admissions Service) entry student nurses. The key differences are:

- RDNAs must complete 2300 hours of supernumerary practice. Any hours in practice where they are working as an employee do not count as practice hours.
- RDNAs also have an end point assessment (EPA) to meet the requirements of the Institute of Apprenticeships at the end of their programme.

For nursing associates Part 1: Standards framework for nursing and midwifery education and Part 2: Standards for student supervision and assessment that were discussed above, apply to them equally. However, they have a different set of Programme standards: Standards for pre-registration nursing associate programmes and different proficiencies: Standards of proficiency for registered nursing associates. If you have nursing associate students in your workplace then it is important to look at their proficiencies. You will find that there are a lot of similarities to the pre-registration nursing standards but there are differences, with only five platforms and a reduced number of skills in the skills annexes. However, it is important to note that a nursing associate is a very specific role that was designed for healthcare providers in England only. They *bridge the gap between healthcare assistants and registered nurses* (NMC, 2020), are generic roles who gain experience across all four fields of practice and across the lifespan and can register with the NMC on successful completion of their programme. Apprentice nursing associates also have an EPA at the end of their 2-year programme to meet the requirements of the Institute of Apprenticeship standards for nursing associates.

Action Points

1. Find out how practice supervisors and practice assessors are prepared in your organisation.
2. Keep reflections on your experience of supporting students in practice and any feedback you received from them or on your performance in supporting them as evidence for your revalidation.
3. Look at the NMC's *Supporting Information on Standards for Student Supervision and Assessment* (SISSSA) hub on their website for more information and guidance on your role (web link at the end of this chapter).
4. Look at the NMC skills annexes in the *Standards of proficiency for registered nurses* and *Standards of proficiency for nursing associates* and consider which skills could be achieved in your area of practice.

USEFUL WEBSITES

Health Education and Improvement Wales: Once for Wales 2020: https://heiw.nhs.wales/programmes/once-for-wales-2020/

NHS Education for Scotland: https://www.nes.scot.nhs.uk/our-work/nursing-and-midwifery-practice-education/

Northern Ireland Practice and Education Council for Nursing and Midwifery: https://nipec.hscni.net/

Nursing and Midwifery Council: Standards for nurses https://www.nmc.org.uk/standards/standards-for-nurses/

Nursing and Midwifery Council: Standards for nursing associates: https://www.nmc.org.uk/standards/standards-for-nursing-associates/

Nursing and Midwifery Council: Supporting information on standards for student supervision and assessment: https://www.nmc.org.uk/supporting-information-on-standards-for-student-supervision-and-assessment/

Chapter 3

Preparing for Students

Chapter Outline

INTRODUCTION

It is a requirement by the NMC that 'there are suitable systems, processes, resources and individuals in place to ensure safe and effective coordination of learning within practice learning environments' (NMC, 2018b, p. 5). This means that it is important that as a practice supervisor or assessor that you and your colleagues are prepared for students before they arrive if you want them to have a safe, effective, and (importantly) a positive learning experience. Good preparation also means that the experience will be far less stressful for the student, yourself and the staff you work with, as everything will be in place for the student and everyone will feel appropriately prepared to support them. Unfortunately, it is not uncommon for students to find that no one is expecting them on their first day and this affects the student's confidence that the placement will be able or willing to provide them with appropriate learning opportunities and that they are going to be sufficiently supported. This chapter will explore the areas you should consider when preparing for a student's arrival, how to identify and mitigate potential problems, and will look at specific aspects of preparation such as information packs and off-duty considerations that can make each student placement a positive experience.

BEFORE THE STUDENT ARRIVES

The NMC requirement that pre-registration nursing students spend 50% of their programme on practice placements can result in some placement areas having a constant flow of students through the door. For some placement providers the students will come from multiple universities and they may all be at different stages in their programme. This means that each student will have different learning needs and require different levels of support. For many staff, having students in their practice area on a regular basis can end up feeling like it is just part of the daily routine. However, it is important to consider the student's perspective in all this. While you may tend to see them as 'just another student', they will arrive in your practice area with all the fears and anxieties that are entirely normal when entering a new environment. From the student's point of view, the first day of placement is vitally important, as it sets the scene for the whole placement (Tremayne & Hunt, 2019). If a student feels welcomed straight away, this ensures the best possible start and they will be more likely to maintain a positive outlook throughout the entire placement. There is just no substitute for a student going home after the first day thinking 'I love my ward/unit/clinic/day centre'. However, if a student gets off to a bad start, they will feel very demoralised and even more anxious about the weeks to come.

Student Expectations

Every student that commences a placement in your practice area will arrive with a certain set of expectations. These expectations will be based partly on previous experiences, partly on the information they may have received from other students and/or the preparation for practice sessions provided by the university, and partly on any previous contact they may have had with your practice area. This may have been in the form of a pre-placement visit or by looking at an online profile of the placement. If a student's expectations are not met, they may begin the placement with a negative mindset. On the other hand, meet these expectations and the placement is far more likely to be successful for both student and the staff working with them (Tremayne & Hunt, 2019).

Likewise, you will also have expectations about the student. If your student meets these expectations on the first day, this will no doubt influence your opinion regarding them. If they do not meet your expectations, then you may have concerns about how their time with you will pan out. Yet the expectations that students and practice supervisors and assessors may have of each other may be based on unreasonable or unrealistic assumptions or misunderstandings that can only be resolved through honest and open communication. This type of communication must take place before the placement begins, and as such, is a vital part of pre-placement preparation. This means that before a student arrives in your practice area you will need to have prepared specifically for their arrival. This will take planning, co-ordination and communication with your whole team. Some practice areas have a dedicated person who takes the lead in preparing for the arrival of students and ensures all resources are in place, including staff. Whilst the initial activities may require time, once systems and processes are in place, they can save you time for each future student being placed with you, and in addition save time and stress by ensuring there are no misunderstandings or breakdowns in communication that lead to complications later on in the placement.

IS YOUR PRACTICE AREA PREPARED?

Let us assume that a student nurse is starting their placement in your practice area next week. Now stop and think for a moment. Would you be prepared? Before you consider the answer, have a look and reflect on the following questions:

1. Is there any particular preparation that is routinely undertaken by your clinical area before a student arrives?
2. Is there a system in place that ensures that the staff in your area are prepared for students' arrival?
3. Is there a system for allocating a practice supervisor and practice assessor to each student allocated in advance of their arrival?
4. Do you have prepared information or guidance for students placed with you?
5. Are all staff fully informed about the programmes that students allocated to them are undertaking and what they will need to learn?

If you have answered *yes* to all of these questions, then your practice area is well on the way to preparing for students. Hopefully this chapter can help to identify ways that you may be able to develop and improve on your current practices. However, if you have answered *no* to any of the above questions, then it is possible that your area is not fully prepared for students and further preparation is needed.

Without specific systems to prepare for students in place, it is possible that students will be faced with a 'lucky dip' of experiences on their first day. They may be lucky and be welcomed and have a positive experience; however, with little or no preparation they may end up feeling unwelcome and unwanted, which can impact negatively on their learning. This may have happened to you as a student; if not, consider how you would have felt on your first day on your current job if you had turned up and no one was expecting you? Unfortunately this scenario is not uncommon. Without good preparation and an agreed plan that all staff are aware of, a student's first day can easily become a poor experience for them. Sometimes it goes wrong due to unforeseen circumstances, such as low staffing numbers or key staff being absent due to sickness; however, often it reflects poor preparation, poor communication or a lack of a contingency plan. Unfortunately, while it is never the intention of staff to not be prepared, it is a common occurrence which students write about in their evaluations of practice. It is also seen in the National Student Survey they complete in their final year. If a student's first experience of practice is of feeling unwanted and unwelcome, then some work will be needed to re-establish trust and ensure that the student feels confident that all will go well.

! A noticeboard in the staff room with the start and end dates and names of students who have been allocated to your practice area, with named practice assessors and supervisors identified for each, is a simple visual reminder of when students are starting and will show the students that the area is prepared for them.

WHAT CAN GO WRONG?

When problems arise at the start of a placement this is often due to a lack of preparation by the placement; it can also, however, include poor preparation by the student.

The Ideal First Day

Let's look at a placement from a student's perspective. Imagine you are about to walk through the door on your first day of a new placement. What do you think would be the best-case scenario for what you would like to happen next? There are some ideas listed below to get you started, but you might like to add in your own ideas based on your own experiences. You were a student once too, so you can use this opportunity to reflect on your own experiences when you were a student nurse.

Examples of best practice for a student's first day are:

- The student is met by their practice supervisor and practice assessor and welcomed by name – it is clear they are expected.
- The practice supervisor introduces the student to the staff on duty that day, explaining who they are (including administrative staff and members of the multidisciplinary team as appropriate).
- The student is shown where they can store their bag/coat, etc.

- The student is welcomed into the team working that day and encouraged to join in at the handover/team meeting.
- The student is given a tour of the area.

The list above represents what would be the ideal first day for any student. Unfortunately, first days do not always go this way, and students find they are not expected or just left to find their own way round the placement with no idea as to who anyone is.

The Unprepared Student

All students are told that they should make contact with their placement in advance, as part of their preparation for practice. Sometimes the student may not know where they are going until the last minute, either because the university has had difficulty finding an appropriate placement or the original placement has fallen through at the last minute. This leaves little time for the student to make contact with their placement in advance. Sometimes it can also be difficult for the student to get in contact with the right person on placement before they start, either by phone or by dropping in on the off chance that someone will be able to help them, even more so if their impending arrival has not been communicated to the nursing team. A student who has failed to make contact in advance for whatever reason will be walking into their placement on the first day totally unprepared, which is not a good start for the student or their practice supervisor or assessor.

The Unprepared Placement

Once again, imagine you are about to walk through the door on your first day of a new placement. However, this time you are required to reflect on the following. What is the worst-case scenario for what might happen next? Just as in the ideal first-day scenario above there are suggestions to get you started; add in your own ideas based on your own experiences.

Examples of things that can go wrong and lead to a poor first day for a student are:

- No one greets the student, no one can find their name on any list – it is clear that they are not expected.
- No one introduces the student to any of the staff on that day and no one seems to know who their practice supervisor or assessor should be or if anyone was designated to welcome them that day.
- The student is told that there is nowhere for them to put their belongings as all lockers and cupboards are full.
- The student sits in on handover/team meeting but feels that they are in the way, as no one includes them in the discussion or checks that they understand the terms being used.
- After handover staff leave the room and the student is left alone, unsure what to do next.

The scenarios above are all real experiences described by students on their first day. Whilst problems can always arise and the best laid plans can go wrong, as a practice supervisor or assessor you should be striving to create a positive experience and to enable students to feel welcomed on their first day. Without planning how to achieve this, the student is more likely to experience elements of the worst-case scenario rather than the best-case scenario. It is important therefore to think through what potential problems might occur, so systems can be put in place to prevent problems before they arise.

If you are expecting a student and they have not made contact before they are due to start it is worth contacting the university to ask if the student is still coming or if there are any problems. Sometimes there is a last-minute change and the information has not reached you, or the student has had problems getting through on the phone, but sometimes the student simply has not made contact. If it is the latter, then the university can prompt the student to contact you. Simply hoping they will turn up leaves both you and the student unprepared for that first day.

> ! When planning for a student's arrival, identify all the elements you would like to happen on the first day and then plan step by step what needs to be done to achieve each of those elements, including back-up plans, so it is not dependent on one person to ensure success.

CREATING A POSITIVE LEARNING ENVIRONMENT

Before any student arrives in your clinical area it is important to ensure that you have prepared a learning environment that is suitable for them. Students are not with you just to complete a set number of hours. The purpose of a practice placement is for students to learn while they are with you, through practising skills, developing and applying their knowledge and role modelling the professional behaviours of staff. It is your responsibility therefore to ensure that your area as a practice placement is a suitable environment for students to learn in and from.

Learning Opportunities

Start by asking yourself these questions:

1. What opportunities are there for students to learn in my area?
2. What activities do we undertake that students might learn from and through?

No doubt you will be able to identify a number quite quickly. For example, drug rounds, wound dressings, patient assessment and observation, talking with service users, helping individuals to manage their anxiety, undertaking risk assessments, working alongside other health and social care professionals to name a few. Each of these activities are potential learning opportunities. A learning opportunity is any event or activity that exists in a placement area that a student might learn something from either by taking part or observing. Consider the potential learning opportunities available to students. Hopefully, you will have identified a range of learning opportunities for students. It is likely that there will be opportunities that are suitable for students at different stages of their programme, that is first-year, second-year and third-year students. For example, cannulation may not be relevant for a first year, but all first years need to learn how to undertake a basic assessment of a patient or service user. It would be worthwhile to indicate in your list of learning opportunities the level of the student that each opportunity is most applicable to. This will help you decide the different groups of students that can and should be encouraged to undertake their clinical experience in your area.

> ! If your area has a student welcome folder, or information provided online, consider including a list of the learning opportunities and learning experiences available to students. Students will find this a valuable resource, and it will reassure them that they will be encouraged to learn as much as possible while on their placement.

The Non-learning Environment

It is always difficult to plan learning experiences for students as the pace of change can be rapid and so often difficult to plan ahead. However, thinking through what opportunities are commonly available and what are appropriate for the students that are allocated to you, can be planned for. If your placement area has been supporting students for a number of years, then it is best practice to regularly reconsider whether any of the learning opportunities have changed. The new *Standards of proficiency*, one each for pre-registration nurses, midwives and nursing associates, have expanded the range of skills they are expected to achieve, so you may find it helpful to look at the standards of proficiency on the NMC website relevant to the students allocated to you (https://www.nmc.org.uk/standards/). Healthcare is in a constant state of change, it is not unreasonable to assume that the learning opportunities available to students will also be likely to fluctuate and that opportunities that were once rare will start to become commonplace. Thus, don't be tied just to the skills listed by the NMC.

In addition to the NMC standards you will find it helpful to look at the practice assessment document (PAD) that sets out the learning students are required to achieve in practice. Most universities will make copies of these documents available to you through your organisation's intranet, the university's own practice education website or a website for universities and placement providers across a geographic area. For example, some regions across England have web-sites with resources for practice supervisors and assessors of nurses and nursing associates including copies of the PAD being used in that region, such as:

- The Pan London Practice Learning Group (PLPLG)
- The Midlands, Yorkshire and East of England Practice Learning Group (MYEPLG)

Scotland, Wales and Northern Ireland also have websites to support staff in practice, with key documents available, such as:

- NHS Education for Scotland
- Once for Wales 2020
- Northern Ireland Practice and Education Council for Nursing and Midwifery: Future Nurse Future Midwife.

If you cannot find a copy of the PADs used by students allocated to your area, contact your Link Lecturer or member of staff from your local university and ask for a copy. Knowing what is expected of the students you are support-ing will help you to plan the types of learning experiences that will help them to achieve their skills and proficiencies. Having considered the range of learning opportunities that are available for students in your practice area you may now wish to consider how this information can be collated for students to use.

Another aspect to consider is which of the learning opportunities are more suitable to particular groups of students. Practice is fast changing and as a con-sequence the range of learning opportunities may change. The audit undertaken by the university should pick this up but if you believe that your area is more suitable for a specific group of students then you should discuss this with your manager and/or contact the university to discuss appropriate student allocation. Matching the learning opportunities to the right students will enable more suc-cessful experiences for all involved.

PERSONAL PREPARATION

Having considered whether your area is prepared for students, the next step is to ensure that you are personally prepared for your role and responsibilities, be it as a practice supervisor or as a practice assessor. Chapter 2 discussed the roles of practice supervisors and practice assessors so do re-read it to remind yourself of the expectations of the roles and preparation needed.

Am I Competent?

The NMC sets the professional standard that is expected of both practice assessors and practice supervisors in their Standards for student supervision and assessment (SSSA) standards (NMC, 2018b). As part of this professional accountability, you are expected to be familiar with you role and responsibilities as a supervisor or assessor, have been appropriately prepared and practice assessors should also have an understanding of the student's programme and the proficiencies they need to achieve. The SSSA set out these responsibilities and whether you are acting as a supervisor or an assessor you are also expected to have up-to-date knowledge and experience of the areas of practice that you are supervising or assessing the student in.

The NMC revalidation process (NMC, 2019a) ensures that you keep your knowledge and skills up to date. Reflecting on feedback from students you have supported or your experiences of preparing for students, supporting them, giving feedback and, if a practice assessor, assessing students are all valuable experiences to reflect on when you have your revalidation discussion with your confirmer. You can use revalidation to demonstrate that you have adequately prepared for your role. In essence, all these measures are there to ensure that practice supervisors and assessors are competent to undertake their role in supporting students on clinical placement.

Do I Understand the Nursing and Midwifery Council Requirements?

The NMC Standards for nurses and nursing associates include the proficiencies that each student is expected to achieve by the end of their programme. The standards are readily available on the NMC website at https://www.nmc.org.uk/standards and they will provide you with an overview of the requirements for student nurses and nursing associates as well as Return to Practice and prescribing programmes. In the next chapter we will look at what students are required to learn whilst in practice in more detail; however, for now, you should use the NMC Standards as a guide in your preparation for students allocated to your practice area.

Do I Understand the Students Programme?

If you are expecting students in your practice area, then part of your preparation is to ensure that you are up to date with the current programme requirements for the students allocated to you. At the very least you will need to have a general understanding of the taught content of the programme, the current educational level of the students that will be allocated, and the purpose of the practice placement they will be undertaking with you. For example, in their first year student nurses are learning about the fundamentals of nursing care and the professional role of the nurse. A mental health student may be allocated to a medical or surgical ward to learn about physical health skills. Nursing associate students are allocated across all fields of practice. Not only will this knowledge aid you in planning learning experiences during the placement, it will also assist you in determining expectations for competence. This information should be a part of your preparation before students arrive in your clinical area.

If you are unsure about the programme the students allocated are undertaking, then there are various ways of finding it out. The university will have provided your practice area with information regarding their students' programme. This may be in the form of a website or a handbook. In addition, it may also be covered during face-to-face updates. If you have students from a number of different universities, keeping abreast of all the different courses can be challenging, so your first meeting with the student is important to enable you to find out what they have studied so far on their programme.

> ! Consider developing some resources for your clinical area with the support of the Link Lecturer. It can be a fast way to access materials and information supplied by the university on the students' programme. These could be posters, flyers or electronic documents or weblinks to each university's website that have information for placement providers.

Do I Understand my Accountability and Responsibility as a Practice Supervisor or Practice Assessor?

A vital part of your personal preparation for students is ensuring that you are familiar with and understand your professional accountability and responsibility as an NMC registrant. The SSSA state that

'all nurses, midwives and nursing associates contribute to practice learning in accordance with The Code' *(NMC, 2018b standard 1.11)*.

The Code specifically states that you must:

'9.4 support students' and colleagues' learning to help them develop their professional competence and confidence' *and*

'20.8 act as a role model of professional behaviour for students and newly qualified nurses, midwives and nursing associates to aspire to' *(NMC, 2018a)*.

The above make clear the expectations of the NMC with regards to your responsibility as a registrant towards students, regardless of whether you are a designated practice supervisor or practice assessor.

Do I Know How to Access Support?

Supporting students can sometimes be a challenging experience. Prior to a student arriving in your practice area you should make yourself aware of the support mechanisms available to you with regards to your role. The support available to you may come in a variety of forms. Most universities supply placement providers with a wide range of paper and electronic resources that can be used by staff who support students in practice. Such resources may include the following:

- Copies of the practice assessment documents
- A guide to using the practice assessment document
- Newsletters
- Key policies relevant to student learning in practice
- Online MOOCS or workshop materials.

In addition, there is a network of people who may be contacted for support during a student's placement. These may include:

- Link Lecturers
- Programme leaders
- Practice educators/facilitators
- Academic assessors.

Very often the lecturers will be involved in visits to the clinical area at scheduled times or provide a drop-in clinic or surgery. In addition, your organisation may also provide resources or people who can support you in your role. These may include:

- Placement facilitators
- Managers
- Practice educators
- Lecturer practitioners.

It is your responsibility to ensure that you are aware of all the support mechanisms available to you prior to students commencing clinical placement. You should be aware of what the specific resources available to you are, who to contact, and how to contact them before students arrive.

PLANNING FOR STUDENTS

Before students arrive in your practice area there needs to be some specific planning undertaken to ensure everyone is ready for their arrival. Remember our example of the 'ideal first day'? This ideal can only be reached if everyone works together and there are clear channels of communication.

How Do I Know When to Expect Students?

It is the responsibility of the university to allocate students to their practice placement, although this is always done through collaboration with a key contact in the organisation. The allocation will have been agreed in advance with this key person who is responsible for student allocations within your organisation.

Before a student's arrival in the clinical area the university is required to inform each placement of the following:

- When the student will be arriving
- The name of the student
- The length of placement
- The course the student is on (they could be a BSc or MSc/PGDip student, a nursing associate or a student on a return to practice programme)
- The students' stage on their programme (first year, second year, etc.)
- Any study days or other activities planned during their placement.

The information regarding a student's arrival will be passed on through a letter, an email or is accessible to the placement via a designated website. Each practice area will have been informed by the university how they can expect to receive this information and what they are required to do to access it. However, it is the responsibility of 'somebody' in each placement to ensure that this information is accessed, and then shared amongst the staff so that everyone is aware of who to expect and when they are expected. If students arrive unexpectedly in your clinical area, then there are three possible explanations for this.

The most common explanation is that while 'someone' should be aware of a student's arrival, the system has failed in some way and either 'nobody' has accessed this information or the information has not been passed on. In either case, best practice in this circumstance is for this information to be checked as soon as possible against the records supplied by the university to the placement. While this information is being checked it is very important that the student is welcomed and the disruption minimised. Remember that the student will be feeling very nervous anyway, and if they are made to feel unwanted this will only exacerbate their anxiety.

It may be that the university has inadvertently forgotten to pass on this information, or the information is sitting in an unread email. Once again, someone in the clinical area should check with the university to ascertain if the student has definitely been allocated to them. It is for this reason that knowing who and how to contact the university is a vital part of preparing for students. Again, while the information is being checked the student should be welcomed and made to feel at ease.

The last possibility is that the student has turned up to the wrong place. This is not common but can occur if the student is new to your organisation or has had limited experience of clinical placements. If it is found that they are in the wrong placement then redirect them to the correct place if it is within your organisation or refer them back to the university so the correct placement location can be identified.

> ! A student notice board or resource folder is a great way to advertise when students are expected. If they are kept up to date, staff can be easily informed and students will feel welcome and wanted.

How Many Students Should I Expect?

The educational audit undertaken of your placement determines how many students can be allocated at any one time, what types of students and at what stage of their programme. The university uses this information to plot placements for the year in conjunction with the lead for placements in your organisation. This number is used to ensure that students are distributed as evenly and fairly as possible and that there are enough practice assessors and supervisors at any one time to facilitate the student numbers allocated to the placement. If your placement capacity changes due to changes in staffing levels, then it is important that the university is informed as soon as possible. The number of students you receive, and the frequency of students, will be directly related to the audit information that has been supplied to the university.

Pre-placement Visits

The university is required to provide advanced notice of the students allocated to your placement and will inform the student once the placement confirms they can support them. This should be at least 4 to 6 weeks before they are due to start. Students will be encouraged to arrange a pre-placement visit, which can facilitate the following:

- Introductions and building a rapport
- Orientation to the layout of the practice area
- Location of emergency equipment
- The placement policy on students answering the phone
- Confirmation of shift times, shift patterns and travel arrangements
- An induction booklet to the placement and any prereading that may help them to prepare (this can be hard copy or sent by email)
- Names of their practice supervisor and practice assessor
- Discussion of any adjustments the student may need (see Chapter 10).

A pre-placement visit should be viewed as an informal opportunity for you to meet with the student. Very often it can be arranged over the telephone or via email and does not have to use a lengthy period of time. If you can, try to provide your student with their off-duty for at least the first week of placement so that they can plan both travel and home commitments and confirm with them where they should report to on the first day of their placement. If there are any special considerations that the student may not be aware of—for example, parking arrangements—then ensure your student is informed. Taking the time to meet a student prior to the placement will pay dividends in the long term: not only will they arrive on the placement feeling welcome, but they will also already feel that you care about them and their learning experience. If a pre-placement visit is not possible, then to ease the student's transition to the placement (especially if it is their first placement) consider asking the student to attend after handover on their first day where they can be orientated to the placement. This can reduce the stress of dealing with handover, where they can be overwhelmed with the amount of information provided and the number of new people they meet.

Allocating the Practice Supervisor and Practice Assessor

One of the key features of preparing for student placement involves allocating a practice assessor and at least one practice supervisor to each student in advance of the placement commencing. Not only is this best practice from a practical point of view, it is also a requirement by the NMC that each student has a nominated practice assessor. It also ensures that some thought has been put into the capacity of the staff allocated to facilitate the student's learning and assessment for the full placement period. For example, it is good to ensure that one of them is available on the student's first day and that this person does not have any extended leave during the student's placement, such as holidays or study leave. Sadly, it is not unusual for students to find out that the person allocated to be their practice assessor is going to be on leave during a crucial stage of the student's placement, or their practice assessor has had to take sick leave. This can result in the student not having their PAD completed. If this occurs on the final placement at the end of a programme part (or year) they may not be able to progress to the next part of the programme or even qualify on time. Whilst the student has a responsibility to let someone on their placement or at the university know this has occurred, some students feel quite vulnerable and do not like to create a fuss.

> ! A designated lead for students in a placement (or group of placements) can ensure someone has oversight of the student experience and can pick up where problems are arising quickly.

If the allocation of the practice supervisor and assessor is not planned, then this can end up being a rushed decision with little thought put into whether they will be able to support the student through the length of their placement. In these circumstances facilitation of learning and assessment may be problematic, with a poor experience for students and staff.

Planning the Off-duty

The only way to guarantee that you are able to supervise your student adequately while they are on their practice placement is to ensure that they are matched to the off-duty with at least one practice supervisor as much as possible, with some shifts also occurring when their nominated practice assessor is also on duty. In working identical shifts you will have the maximum opportunity of facilitating learning experiences and also give yourself a chance to give them feedback on their progress. You will also be able to accurately record the number of hours they have attended on placement, with sicknesses and absences tracked carefully. Both you and your student will benefit equally from this arrangement. It works especially well if the practice supervisor and assessor are allocated prior to the placement beginning, as this also ensures that they are able to greet the student on their first day of placement. The NMC requires that students make themselves available for the full range of 24/7 shifts across weekdays and weekends so that they can experience all aspects of patient care (although night duty on their very first placement is not advisable). This requirement should make it a simple process to match a student's off-duty with you for the entire placement period. It will also have the added benefit of ensuring that the practice supervisor and practice assessor will be available for the full placement experience, and that a booked holiday or period of study leave has not been forgotten.

There is no expectation that a student is on the same shift with the same practice supervisor every day. The level of supervision will depend on the student's learning needs and stage of their programme. Students may work with a number of different practice supervisors during their placement. What is essential is that practice supervisors and practice assessors communicate, so that there is regular feedback on student progression. This may be simply speaking with each other or feedback can be documented in the student's PAD. It may be that it is not possible for one specific practice supervisor to work every shift with the student; therefore identifying additional practice supervisors who can support the student is important. Box 3.1 shows two different off-duty rotas for the first 2 weeks of a student's placement.

BOX 3.1 Example Shift Rotas

Rota A

	M	T	W	Th	F	S	S	M	T	W	Th	F	S	S
Student	LD		LD			LD	LD	LD		LD			LD	
Practice Supervisor A			LD	LD	LD			LD		LD	LD			LD
Practice Supervisor B		LD		LD		LD		LD		LD			LD	LD
Practice Assessor		LD		LD	LD			LD		LD		LD		LD

Rota B

	M	T	W	Th	F	S	S	M	T	W	Th	F	S	S
Student	LD		LD			LD	LD	LD		LD			LD	
Practice Supervisor A	LD		LD		LD	LD	LD	LD						LD
Practice Supervisor B		LD		LD		LD		LD		LD			LD	LD
Practice Assessor	LD	LD			LD			LD	LD		LD		LD	LD

In rota A, neither of the practice supervisors or the practice assessor are on duty on the student's first day and there are several days when the student does not have either of their nominated practice supervisors on duty with them at all. A junior student may well feel lost and uncared for if no one else steps in to support them. You will also notice that the practice assessor is not on duty at all during the student's first 2 weeks. They do, however, have some shifts with the student's practice supervisors and so can get feedback on the student's first few days from them. Whilst it is not essential for the practice assessor to have all the same shifts as the student, it is important that key points to meet up are planned during the student's placement. Students are very anxious about meeting up with their practice assessor, so seeing them early on in their placement, even if just to say hello and let them know how they will be supported and assessed through the placement, can reduce that anxiety considerably. It is also important to note that if no one is allocated to supervise the student on their first day that their induction to the placement may not take place, which could lead to health and safety issues if the student does not know their way around the placement and where key equipment can be found.

In rota B, a nominated practice supervisor and practice assessor are on duty on the student's first day. The student has most of the same shifts as practice supervisor A, but when they are not on the same shifts a second supervisor has been identified for them. The practice assessor is also on the same shift at the end of the second week, so allowing them an opportunity to catch up on the student's progress.

A word of caution here; some students may have very specific requests around their off-duty, and whilst some flexibility is reasonable, they are on placement to learn and need to undertake a range of shifts. If they dictate when they can attend practice, this can lead to minimal or patchy supervision during the placement. It is an NMC requirement that all students are supervised in practice and whilst the level of supervision will depend on their learning needs and stage in the programme (NMC, 2018b), close working in the early stages is helpful in determining what level of supervision the student needs. Students are not simply on the placement to complete a set number of hours. If you have a student who makes special requests as a result of personal circumstances or outside obligations that affect their learning experience and the ability of staff to supervise them, then seek advice from the university. If they are an apprenticeship student then their employer also needs to be informed. In some cases these specific requests may be due to reasonable adjustments the student requires, which we will discuss in Chapter 10, but sometimes the request may not be reasonable.

! Aim to allocate each student the same off-duty as their practice supervisor(s) and some shifts with their practice assessor before the placement begins. This will ensure that any difficulties the student has in attending placement for the full range of shifts is identified early and the university can be contacted for advice. You could consider using the pre-placement visit to finalise these details so the student can prepare for their shift pattern before the placement begins.

PREPARATION OF RESOURCES

It is quite common for placement areas to provide students with a range of resources that may be used prior to or during a practice placement to familiarise themselves with the environment. Generally these consist of three different types of resources: online student information, student information packs/folder, and/or student noticeboards. This section explores these different types of resources and how they may be used as part of the preparation for students.

Online Placement Profiles

Some universities (and some placement providers) provide students with placement information that can be accessed online. The information may be categorised into various sections, and may include some or all of the following features:

- Brief summary of the area and the type of patients/service users that students will care for
- Contact details for the clinical area
- Shift times
- Travel directions
- Glossary of important terms used in the area
- Key documents related to the speciality, such as National Institute for Health and Care Excellence (NICE) guidelines
- Organisational policies
- University policies for the placement.

In addition, there is often an opportunity for a clinical area to provide a summary of their specialty and the types of patients/service users cared for in these profiles. Placement areas may also have the opportunity of outlining learning opportunities for students and specific preparation/revision that students should do prior to commencing the placement. If these profiles are used in your organisation, then you could consider forming a group of staff who take responsibility for updating the online information. Spending 5 to 10 minutes every month checking that the information provided is relevant will ensure that students are given up-to-date information prior to commencing placement.

Student Information Packs/Folders

Many placement areas provide a student pack or folder for students to access during the placement. These can be a valuable source of information. Many students find that resources like this are invaluable as an aid to their orientation to the clinical environment. A good starting point is to consider the following:

- A profile of the staff working in the area – a 'who's who', including the multidisciplinary team
- Contact details of relevant people – for example, Link Lecturers

- A brief description of the type of placement/specialty
- Learning opportunities for students (you may wish to split these into opportunities for first, second, and third years)
- A glossary of key terms
- Some recommended further reading that is related to the specialty.

Unless there is some specific reason for doing so, try not to include too much information in a student folder. Point them to where key information is available; this ensures they can access the most up-to-date information. For example, organisations now provide policies via their intranet sites, and so the student folder should contain details of how they may access these policies, including usernames and passwords if required. Asking students what they found useful in the folder or what was missing that needs adding is a valuable way of ensuring it meets the needs of current and future students.

Student Noticeboards

Many practice areas allocate a specific section or separate noticeboard for student information. This is a great idea and can be very useful for students if it contains good, relevant and up-to-date information. However, because a noticeboard is very visual it can very quickly become a negative rather than a positive if it is not kept up to date or if too much information is on there. If you are going to have a student noticeboard then you could consider providing the following information:

- Link Lecturer details and availability
- Details of student drop-in clinics or student surgeries available locally
- Upcoming talks, lectures, teaching sessions within your organisation that students may be able to attend
- Names of students, their nominated practice assessors and dates when initial, mid and final interviews are due.

Remember that a student noticeboard does not have to be huge; it is far better to have a small amount of relevant information than vast quantities of out-of-date information. Again, asking students for feedback is a good way of ensuring it meets their needs.

! If you have never had a student noticeboard before, start very small and build up slowly. Try starting with an area no bigger than A1 and make sure that someone is prepared to review the noticeboard regularly to ensure that the information is current, useful and interesting.

Updating Student Information

No matter what resource is being used in your area to provide information for students, it will have little value if it is not kept up to date. Someone specific in your clinical area will need to be designated with the responsibility of maintaining and updating the information for any resource you have. Maintaining student resources must also happen as part of the preparation for students, so it will need to be constantly monitored.

GETTING STUDENT PREPARATION RIGHT

No matter how much preparation you may have done for a student's placement there will always be occasions when somehow the system falls down. If you have not already done so it may be useful to develop a checklist or guide to areas that need to be regularly monitored to ensure that your area is prepared for students. Making this a part of your staff management routine can ensure that facilitating students runs as smoothly as possible. Box 3.2 provides an example of a student preparation checklist. While there is no guarantee that a checklist will prevent all problems, it will assist in troubleshooting the most

---

BOX 3.2 Checklist for Preparing for Students

Preparation for students checklist	Yes/no
Are there enough practice supervisors for the number of students we have agreed to support?	
Are there enough practice assessors for the number of students we have agreed to support?	
Are the practice supervisors and assessors up to date and prepared to support the student numbers agreed?	
Is there a process for finding out when students are arriving and is there a process to communicate this to everyone?	
Is a named practice assessor allocated prior to the student starting the placement?	
Is at least one practice supervisor allocated prior to the student starting the placement?	
Are the practice supervisor and student rostered to work together?	
Are the practice supervisor and student rostered together on the first day?	
Do the practice supervisor/assessor have any booked leave during the student's time with you and if so is a plan in place to ensure this will not have a negative impact on the assessment process for the student?	
Is there a named contact at the university if there are any issues that arise?	
Is there a process in place to ensure any student resources are kept up to date?	

common areas where student preparation may be overlooked. Get this right and the placement can start under the best possible circumstances.

In this chapter we have discussed many aspects of preparing for students coming to a practice area. We have looked at personal preparation and also preparation from the perspective of the practice environment itself. While a whole chapter has been dedicated to the issue of preparing for students, the fact is that most of the issues addressed are not time-consuming or costly once the initial work has been undertaken. The initial time spent will provide benefits for staff and for the student. Inadequate preparation can lead to a poor student experience and a less than satisfactory experience for the staff supporting them. A placement that has a preparation strategy shows that they value students and the students in turn will value their time there.

APPRENTICE STUDENTS AND NURSING ASSOCIATES

The ideas and suggestions in this chapter also apply to students allocated to you who are Registered Nursing Degree Apprentices, nursing associates, or return-to-practice students. Apprentice students who are allocated to a placement where they are not employed will be supernumerary and so treated no differently from any other students.

Action Points

1. Find out how your workplace is informed about students coming to your practice area and where this information is stored.
2. Develop a strategy for student preparation; prepare yourself and your practice area.
3. Keep yourself up to date with the students' programmes and learning needs.
4. Consider how to welcome students; either by developing welcome packs or noticeboards and arranging pre-placement visits.
5. Develop a 'Student preparation checklist' and ensure it is updated at regular intervals.

Chapter 4

Understanding the Practice Assessment Document

Chapter Outline

INTRODUCTION

The practice assessment document (PAD) and ongoing achievement record (OAR) are core to the student's learning experience in practice. They provide the student and practice supervisors and practice assessors with guidance on the types of learning opportunities that each student needs to experience and identify what the student needs to be assessed on in order to meet the Nursing and Midwifery Council (NMC) proficiencies and programme requirements. They are also communication tools between practice supervisors, practice assessors and academic assessors, as well as other staff in practice who may contribute to the student's learning experiences, including Link Lecturers who meet with the student in practice. The purpose of this chapter is to examine the different sections commonly found in a PAD and the OAR to clarify their purpose and value to you and the student. This can help you to provide positive learning experiences culminating in a fair assessment of the student's achievements. Some countries in the UK have combined the PAD and OAR into one document, whilst other countries have them as two separate documents. The principles of how they are used are the same, regardless. Whilst the term *document* is commonly used, many universities have moved to electronic versions of the document – commonly called *e-PADs*.

BACKGROUND TO THE PRACTICE ASSESSMENT DOCUMENT

At one time each university had its own tool for assessing students in practice. This was not a problem when a placement provider only supported students from one university, but today most placement providers have multiple universities allocating students to them. PADs are invariably lengthy and trying to become familiar with different formats can be difficult for staff supporting students in practice. This can lead to incomplete or inadequate completion of the document which can contribute to the failure to fail of students who are not demonstrating the required values or proficiencies in practice. However, following successful collaborations between groups of universities across each of the four countries of the UK, the adoption of a single document used by multiple universities across geographic regions is now becoming the norm. Examples of these collaborations are:

- In England the document developed by the Pan London Practice Learning Group, called PLPAD 2.0, has been adopted across geographic regions with locally agreed names, for example MYE PAD is used in the Midlands Yorkshire and East of England, the South PAD across the south and southwest of England. One PAD is used for each part (year) of the pre-registration nursing programme. A separate Ongoing Achievement Document (OAR) records the student's journey across their placements across the length of their programme. In addition, there has been collaboration across universities to develop a single PAD for nursing associate programmes.
- Wales, which has a long history of using a single PAD, now has the All Wales PAD and OAR, combining both these elements into one document
- Scotland has the All Scotland Practice Assessment Document
- Northern Ireland has The Northern Ireland Practice Assessment Document (NIPAD): three separate documents which combined equate to an Ongoing Record of Achievement.

Differences in terminology have also been problematic with these documents. Multiple different names have been used, such as:

- Clinical skills book
- Assessment book
- Assessment of practice record
- Practice learning document
- Placement assessment document
- Practice assessment document
- Ongoing achievement record.

The move to single regional documents has seen a common agreement to use the term PAD for the document, which incorporates the assessment of the student against the NMC proficiencies. As noted above, some countries have a separate document called the OAR while others have incorporated this as part of the PAD. The OAR summarises the achievement of the student on each placement and demonstrates *the achievement of proficiencies and skills set out in standards of proficiency for registered nurses* (NMC, 2018c, p. 11) and is used in conjunction with the PAD to provide a comprehensive picture of the student's professional development through each of their placements and across the length of their programme. Many regions/countries have a shared website that all practice partners can access, which holds copies of the PADs, guidance on their use, and other supporting information that practice partners, including practice supervisors and assessors, can use. In addition, most universities will have a website accessible to practice partners with key documentation and guidance to assist practice supervisors and assessors in their role. These may or may not require local practice partners to log in to access course-specific documentation.

One of the challenges with PADs has been that they are lengthy documents; the length is needed to encompass all the elements that need to be assessed. This is even more true if a university has decided to have one document for the whole programme. Traditionally PADs have been a paper or hard copy document, but this format poses a number of challenges, which were summarised by Donaldson et al. (2020) as:

- Illegibility of handwriting
- Incomplete records (missing signatures, proficiencies or other sections missed)
- Poor or limited documentation with regards to feedback and interviews or reflections by the student
- Limited accessibility – staff in practice are reliant on the student bringing the PAD in and staff at the university do not see it until it is submitted at the end of the placement
- Loss or damage to the PAD

- Support limited if the PAD is only seen when the student brings it in, so staff are unaware of what the student needs to do or if they are having difficulties and need support in specific areas
- Submission and moderation is a logistical problem with large documents and cohort sizes
- Verifying authenticity of signatures, especially of practice supervisors/ assessors.

These challenges have led to many universities moving to an electronic version of the PAD.

ELECTRONIC PRACTICE ASSESSMENT DOCUMENTS

Alongside the development of these regional PADs there has also been the development of electronic versions of the PAD, commonly called an e-PAD or ePAD. Each region/university has chosen its own platform, but in general, regardless of the company used, access can be via smartphones, desktop PCs, laptops and tablets. There are a number of benefits to an electronic PAD which in essence are answers to the problems identified above, including:

- Easier to carry around
- Easier to read than the handwritten formats
- Easier to add to and update
- Digital electronic signatures are verifiable
- Accessible online (useful when a student forgets to bring it in to practice)
- Academic staff are able to monitor student progress from a distance as each section and stage of the PAD is completed
- Physical submission isn't required as it is always available to academic staff, so easier to moderate and for external examiners to review
- It cannot be lost like a paper copy can!

However, there are challenges in using an electronic PAD, most commonly around Information technology (IT) access. Some smaller placement providers may not have the level of IT access seen in larger organisations; this is commonly cited as an issue on community placements. There can also be competition where there are limited IT resources which are constantly in use by other staff. This can make it difficult for practice supervisors/assessors who wish to access the e-PAD via a PC on placement if availability is limited. In addition, there are the challenges that exist where there is variability in the level of IT skills of both students and staff.

LAYOUT OF THE PRACTICE ASSESSMENT DOCUMENT

Regardless of whether a PAD is a paper or electronic document, there are key sections within each PAD that are common to all countries and regions.

PADs are developed by universities in conjunction with practice partners and have to be approved by the NMC at the validation of the programme. With the collaborative approach by universities and practice partners to develop a single PAD for a whole region or country, we are now seeing more similarities and less differences in the PADs used by universities across the UK. Some of the key features included within many of the PADs used in the UK at the moment are:

- Student and placement details
- Instructions on how to complete the PAD
- Guidance to practice supervisors/assessors on what to do if there are concerns regarding a student's progress
- Name of the nominated person for the placement and the name of the academic assessor
- Induction checklist
- List of practice supervisors/assessors involved in the student's learning
- Professional values to be achieved on each placement
- The learning outcomes/proficiencies to be achieved
- Clinical skills
- In-point assessments/episodes of care
- Learning contracts/development support plans
- Service user feedback tool
- Reflections by the student
- Feedback to student on progress and final report
- Action plans
- Timesheets.

All PADs are structured to facilitate the student's journey through their placement and the steps of the assessment process. The assessment criteria identify the decreasing levels of supervision required as the student moves from guided supervision to acting independently (see Fig. 4.1). As a result, they will all contain sections for documentation of interviews with students (initial, midpoint, final) which are the essential three stages of the assessment process.

The Introduction

It is very easy to skip the introduction to the PAD, but it is essential reading so that you are clear on what is expected of you. It will include details about the key sections of the PAD, descriptions of the key people involved in completing the PAD, and the roles and responsibilities of each, including the student. It is important to re-read the introduction each time you have a student, as lack of familiarity with the process and what is required of you can lead to errors or omissions when completing the document. Errors and omissions can mean the university requires the student to return to practice to have these errors or omissions corrected, causing

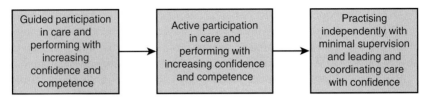

FIG. 4.1   Criteria for assessment through each part of the programme Pan London Practice Assessment Document V2.0. *(Pan London Practice Learning Group, 2019a.)*

the student additional anxiety, although this is less likely with an e-PAD, which requires full completion of required sections to progress to the next one. A common error is where a practice supervisor signs sections in the PAD that only a practice assessor is permitted to sign. The university and practice partners will have made decisions as to who is the best person (practice supervisor or practice assessor) to complete each section of the PAD. This may be detailed in the introduction to the PAD under the roles and responsibilities of practice supervisors and practice assessors; the people who can sign in each section will be clearly identified where it must be a specific person.

Assessment Criteria

The criteria to be used to determine whether a student has achieved their professional values or proficiencies will also be included as part of the introduction. This is a useful guide when making assessment decisions and they are usually provided for each part (stage) of the student's programme, reflecting the stages shown in Fig. 4.1, which show how a student develops their skills, knowledge and values as they progress through each part. Appendix 4.1 shows criteria for achieving or not achieving proficiencies for students across the three levels or parts of a programme. Similar variations of these will be used by all universities, enabling greater consistency in assessment of students across the UK.

Placement Information

Details of the placement and key contacts such as the names of the nominated person for the placement, the Link Lecturer and the academic assessor. The nominated person for the placement is usually the person with overall responsibility for the students on the placement, for example, the Placement Manager, Ward Manager, Team Leader or Service Manager and may also include the Link Lecturer.

Induction Checklist

The induction or orientation checklist is not to be taken lightly, as the process of discussing and confirming each item on the checklist is to ensure the health and safety of both the student and patients/service users by confirming that the student knows where emergency equipment is kept, actions to take in emergency situations, and the location of key policies and procedures. It is also the opportunity to check whether the student requires any reasonable adjustments during their placement, as if any are disclosed the placement has a duty to meet any reasonable adjustments the student requires with respect to disclosure of a disability, additional learning need, or pregnancy. By signing off the induction checklist you are confirming all sections have been discussed and, where actions are required, that they have been completed.

Record of Practice Supervisors/Assessors Involved in the Student's Learning

The names of all practice supervisors and the practice assessor/academic assessor must be recorded. This enables cross-checking if needed to ensure that only appropriately prepared people are undertaking these roles. In a paper document this will also include their signature, which can be used to verify any elements signed in the PAD. In an e-PAD there will be a secure login process and a verification process to ensure that any sections completed are actually done by the named person.

Professional Values

The professional values or professional attitudes and behaviours are based on the NMC *Code* (2018a) and Platform 1 *Being an accountable practitioner* of the NMC *Standards of proficiency for registered nurses* (NMC, 2018d). The professional values are fundamental to becoming a nurse and therefore the students must pass these on each placement. Students will be assessed at midpoint and at the end of each placement. These apply to all four fields of practice.

The Learning Outcomes/Proficiencies to be Achieved

Learning outcomes or proficiencies are based on the NMC *Standards of proficiency for registered nurses* (NMC, 2018d). Depending on the university these may be broad statements which encompass one or more of the NMC proficiencies and/or include the communication and relationship management skills and nursing procedures listed in the two annexes, or they may be the actual proficiency statements from the NMC standards. In either case they state what the student must be able to do, and tend to use words such as *demonstrates*, *utilises*, *collects*, *applies*, *records*, which assists you to understand what the student will need to do to show that they have achieved the proficiency. The outcomes will focus on the knowledge, skills and professional values/behaviours required of the student, with different ones for each part of the programme they are on. These are often completed over the course of the placement and on each occasion the practice assessor has to make the decision on whether the student has achieved the proficiencies to the standard required for the stage of their programme, taking into account their field of practice. For example, an adult field student would be expected to demonstrate a greater level of proficiency at managing blood transfusions than a mental health student, but conversely a mental health student would be expected to demonstrate greater proficiency in using cognitive behavioural therapy techniques than adult or child field students.

Some proficiencies will be very specific, with a clear expectation of what is to be achieved. For example:

Accurately measure weight and height, calculate body mass index and recognise healthy ranges and clinical significance of low/high readings.
(Pan London Practice Learning Group, 2019a).

In this example the expectation of what the student is required to be able to do is very well defined. You are required to verify that the student is competent in a certain skill. Most practice supervisors and assessors would feel quite confident with this type of learning proficiency as it gives explicit direction on what is required. Other proficiencies, however, may be broad and open to interpretation, to enable them to be applied to different care settings. For example:

Demonstrate the skills and abilities required to support people who are emotionally or physically vulnerable.
(All Wales Practice Assessment Document and Ongoing Record of Achievement, 2020).

This has the advantage of not restricting the types of opportunities that must be available for the student and helps to maximise the possibility of the student achieving the standard required. However, these broader proficiencies often pose difficulties for practice supervisors and assessors, as the interpretation of exactly what is required to be learnt and then what evidence the student must produce to demonstrate they have achieved the proficiency may not be immediately apparent.

! If you have difficulties with understanding what the student is required to demonstrate to achieve any proficiency, discuss this with other practice supervisors/assessors in your area or the representative from your university who links to your area.

Clinical Skills

The PAD may also include a list of clinical and communication skills from the annexes in the NMC *Standards of proficiency for registered nurses* (NMC, 2018d), which will need to be achieved by the end of the programme.

In-point Assessments/Episodes of Care

These could be snapshots of patient-centred care activities, or have a specific focus on, for instance, medicines management or teaching and supervising others or leadership and management skills. These will become more complex as the student progresses through each part of the programme. They will therefore require different levels of clinical skill and evidence-based knowledge to be demonstrated by the student for each part of their programme, with increasing levels of proficiency and a knowledge and use of evidence as the student progresses through their programme.

Service User Feedback Tool

It is an NMC requirement that *service users contribute to student assessment* (NMC, 2018e, p. 12). In practice settings a simple Likert scale is commonly used and can be completed by service users or their carers. Whilst this is not seen as a formal part of the assessment process, it is one of many sources of evidence that can be used by the practice supervisor as part of the feedback process to the student and by the practice assessor to contribute to the assessment decision.

Reflections by the Student

PADs may also include sections where students are required to provide evidence of their practice experiences and learning. These may include reflections on their learning, evidence of achieving their proficiencies, or commentaries related to specific practice placement experiences.

Feedback to Student on Their Progress and Final Review

There will be sections throughout the PAD to record feedback to students on their progress. This includes the midpoint and the final review. In addition, there will be opportunities for recording feedback from other health and social care professionals, including feedback on any outreach/out of placement/spoke experiences the student may have undertaken during their placement. Chapter 7 looks at feedback in more detail.

Learning Contracts, Action Plans and Development Support Plans

Most PADs will contain an area for practice supervisors/assessors and students to develop learning contracts/action plans. These are agreed plans between the practice supervisors/assessors and the student, detailing actions to be undertaken to enable the student to achieve specific learning objectives. They should detail who is responsible for each of the agreed actions. These learning contracts may also be called *action plans* or *development support plans*. Chapter 5 will explore the importance of the initial interview, as it is an ideal time to discuss and agree on the plan for learning during the student's time with you. There may be other occasions, such as the midpoint interview, when learning contracts/action plans are also useful. Likewise, action plans are essential if a student is not meeting the expected standard or a new learning opportunity has become available and it is necessary to document an agreement as to how the student will engage with this learning. This is particularly important where the learning opportunity is away from their placement. We will look at the use of learning contracts for students where there are concerns regarding their conduct or competence in more detail in Chapter 8.

What if I Run Out of Space to Document?

When designing a PAD, universities will try to predict the amount of space required by staff in practice to complete the required assessment documentation. If the space given is not sufficient, then it is advisable to contact a Link Lecturer from the university who will discuss the options open to you. As the PAD is a formal assessment document, it is important that all relevant information is recorded, and not simply left out due to a lack of writing space. It may be that you are advised to record additional documentation on headed paper, giving a copy to the student and the Link Lecturer if necessary. One benefit of an electronic PAD is that this is not usually a problem!

Timesheets

These may be part of the PAD, in which case hours must be verified by the practice supervisor/assessor. Some universities may use an on-line process for recording student hours.

DOCUMENTING THE ASSESSMENT PROCESS

Unsurprisingly, the PAD will contain a section where the practice supervisor/ assessor is required to carry out an assessment. Usually this will mean signing or initialling your name against a list of proficiencies or, for electronic PADs, completing the checklist of proficiencies achieved and confirming/validating the areas you have completed. You may be required to decide if proficiencies have been achieved or not achieved; some universities may ask you to grade a student according to a marking grid or predetermined criteria set by the university, although this is less common now. Regular updates by the university and the practice education leads in your organisation should ensure that you are familiar with the process used by your university/ies in assessing students, so this is a vital aspect of your preparation before the student arrives. The PAD should also contain instructions regarding the assessment process required, so you should take the time to read this and clarify any areas that you are unsure about.

Students can be very protective regarding their PADs if they are a paper document, as replacing the document can be quite difficult if lost (this is not a problem with electronic PADs) and the historical record of a student's achievements will be lost. For this reason, students may avoid regularly bringing their PAD to placement for fear of losing or damaging it. Students will have either one PAD that will cover several placements across the year or part of the programme or they may have one PAD for the whole programme (these are more of a problem if lost!).

COMPLETING THE PRACTICE ASSESSMENT DOCUMENT

When completing the PAD it is essential to view the document as being as important as any other nursing record. The NMC Code (2018a) section 10 outlines your responsibility to '*keep clear and accurate records relevant to your practice*'; this is not limited to patient records, so it also includes students' PADs. The Code also reinforces the importance of attributing '*any entries you make in any paper or electronic records to yourself, making sure they are clearly written, dated and timed, and do not include unnecessary abbreviations, jargon or speculation*' (NMC, 2018a, p. 11). Whilst you do not need to include the time of your record in a PAD the rest of the guidance is equally applicable to a student's PAD.

It is essential that you keep statements clear and factual; avoid unspecific generic sentences which could lead to misunderstandings, and sign and date in every space required. Be specific about any agreements with the student; for example, state exactly what the student must do for each proficiency or series of learning opportunities rather than 'we have discussed and agreed what the student needs to do to achieve the proficiencies and professional values'. Remember what you write will be read by other practice supervisors and the practice assessor on the student's current placement with you as well as other practice supervisors/assessors on future placements. The NMC (2018b) *Standards for Student Supervision and Assessment* mean that the student can work with multiple supervisors during a single placement, so see this as not only a record of communication with the student but to all the practice supervisors and the practice assessor involved with the student during their placement. It therefore needs to be constructive and clear for everyone to read.

As stated earlier, the PAD records two essential processes related to the student's placement: the steps taken to ensure the assessment is valid and reliable and the outcome of the assessment. Even if process has been followed, a failure to record this accurately in the PAD can make it very difficult to prove that the correct assessment processes have been followed at a later date. Therefore what you write needs to withstand outside scrutiny. For example, if a student is not making progress in a specific area then this should be discussed with them and documented. If it is not documented you cannot fail them later as there is no evidence that the discussion, agreed actions, and agreed expectations of the student have taken place. This is no different from documenting in patient/service user records, where the mantra is 'if you did not document it, it wasn't done'.

THE ONGOING ACHIEVEMENT RECORD

Where the university uses one separate PAD per part of the programme then there may be a separate OAR. Where they are brought together into one document, that document is also the OAR. Where the OAR is a separate document, the practice assessor will be required to write a summary of the student's achievements and strengths and areas for further development. Think of the OAR as a communication tool between yourself and future practice supervisors and assessors. The OAR can help future practice supervisors and assessors identify areas that the student needs to work on. For example, the practice assessor noted that the feedback in their student's OAR had repeatedly commented on the need for the student to develop their organisation skills. Further discussion elicited that the student had dyslexia and therefore organisation skills were a problem for her. Having identified this as an area to work on, they explored different ways of organising her work for the day; whilst it took her a little longer to complete all the care activities planned, they would all be achieved and in the right priority order. The practice assessor was able to document the progress made and how this was managed. The student felt a real sense of achievement, as at last this aspect of her practice was no longer being consistently commented on and she felt she could move on to focus on and develop new skills.

ASSESSING IN PRACTICE

No matter how committed you are to your role in supporting and developing students, it is essential that you understand a student's PAD. If used correctly, the PAD will guide you and your student through the placement, highlighting where attention is required to the key stages within the assessment process. The PAD will provide a context for the goals of the placement, the opportunities to be explored, and will signpost when and where achievements have to be documented. At the core of every successful practice assessment is a practice supervisor and practice assessor who can understand and use the PAD to inform and direct the assessment process.

Action Points

1. Find out where you can download a copy of the PAD used by your local universities and read through it.
2. Talk to your Link Lecturer and ask them to clarify aspects of the PAD that you may be unfamiliar with.
3. Attend updates for practice supervisors and assessors and discuss with other colleagues your experiences of documenting within the PAD; share good practice.
4. Make a list of commonly used proficiencies that are commonly assessed in your area and ensure all colleagues are following the same interpretation.

Appendix 4.1

Practice Assessment Criteria

'Achieved' must be obtained in all three criteria by the student

PART 1: GUIDED PARTICIPATION IN CARE

Achieved	Knowledge	Skills	Attitude and Values
Yes	Is able to identify the appropriate knowledge base required to deliver safe, person-centred care under some guidance.	In commonly encountered situations is able to utilise appropriate skills in the delivery of person-centred care with some guidance.	Is able to demonstrate a professional attitude in delivering person-centred care. Demonstrates positive engagement with own learning.
No	Is not able to demonstrate an adequate knowledge base and has significant gaps in understanding, leading to poor practice.	Under direct supervision is not able to demonstrate safe practice in delivering care despite repeated guidance and prompting in familiar tasks.	Inconsistent professional attitude towards others and lacks self-awareness. Is not asking questions, nor engaging with own learning needs.

PART 2: ACTIVE PARTICIPATION IN CARE WITH MINIMAL GUIDANCE AND INCREASING CONFIDENCE

Achieved	Knowledge	Skills	Attitude and Values
Yes	Has a sound knowledge base to support safe and effective practice and provide the rationale to support decision making.	Utilises a range of skills to deliver safe, person-centred and evidence-based care with increased confidence and in a range of contexts.	Demonstrates an understanding of professional roles and responsibilities within the multidisciplinary team. Maximises opportunities to extend own knowledge.

Achieved	Knowledge	Skills	Attitude and Values
No	Has a superficial knowledge base and is unable to provide a rationale for care, demonstrating unsafe practice.	With supervision is not able to demonstrate safe practice and is unable to perform the activity and/or follow instructions despite repeated guidance.	Demonstrates lack of self-awareness and understanding of professional role and responsibilities. Is not asking appropriate questions nor engaged with their own learning.

PART 3: LEADS AND COORDINATES CARE

Achieved	Knowledge	Skills	Attitude and Values
Yes	Has a comprehensive knowledge base to support safe and effective practice and can critically justify decisions and actions using an appropriate evidence base.	Is able to safely, confidently and competently manage person-centred care in both predictable and less well recognised situations, demonstrating appropriate evidence-based skills.	Acts as an accountable practitioner in responding proactively and flexibly to a range of situations. Takes responsibility for own learning and the learning of others.
No	Is only able to identify the essential knowledge base, with poor understanding of rationale for care. Is unable to justify decisions made, leading to unsafe practice.	With minimal supervision is not able to demonstrate safe practice despite guidance.	Demonstrates lack of self-awareness and professionalism. Does not take responsibility for their own learning and the learning of others.

Chapter 5

Orientation and the Initial Interview

Chapter Outline

INTRODUCTION

The first week of a student's placement is a crucial time and how this is managed will influence how well the placement goes for the student and the practice supervisors and practice assessor who will be supporting the student during their time with them. The initial interview sets the scene and should have a clear structure to ensure all key areas regarding the student's needs and expectations are covered. The orientation to the placement is also a key requirement as it both helps the student to become familiar with the placement and also meets key health and safety requirements. Planning and preparation for this first stage of the student's learning journey with you is therefore very important and will need to include an understanding of the student's learning needs based upon the practice assessment document (PAD) and any personal objectives and reasonable adjustments they may need to succeed on their placement with you. Knowledge and understanding of how students learn is essential to enable learning opportunities to meet individual learning styles. It is also important that there is an understanding of the requirements of the student's course if the plans for their learning are to meet both student and course requirements.

PREPARING FOR THE ORIENTATION AND INITIAL INTERVIEW

Chapter 3 explored the preparation that should take place before a student arrives in your clinical area. The purpose of thorough preparation is to identify any potential problems that may affect their placement with you and to ensure that the practice placement gets off to the best possible start for both you and your student. As a reminder, here are some key things you need to prepare before the student arrives:

- Student has been allocated a named practice supervisor (minimum of one, but could be more) and a named practice assessor.
- Off-duty has been agreed and aligns with the off-duty for the practice supervisor and/or practice assessor.
- The student's programme and stage on their programme are known.
- Copies of the relevant PADs are available so that staff can consider learning opportunities in advance that align with the PADs.
- If an e-PAD is being used by the student, then all practice supervisors and practice assessors have been prepared to use the e-PAD and have accounts or other requirements such as an NHS email address or private health provider email address in order to access the student's e-PAD.
- Who will undertake the initial meeting and complete the orientation/induction checklist has been established. Ideally having both the practice supervisor and practice assessor present is best, as it ensures that everyone is clear about any plans and expectations. If only one person can attend, it is important to check what has been agreed by the university as to who can undertake the initial interview.

MEETING YOUR STUDENT

If you are properly prepared for your student's arrival, then the initial meeting should be a relaxed and friendly event. Ideally, you will have had contact with the student previously, either through a pre-placement visit or via phone or email. The first meeting is your opportunity to welcome them to the placement area and ensure they feel wanted and welcome. You only have one chance to get this right, so it is really important that this is handled well, as this first meeting will set the tone for the rest of the placement. No matter how much information they may have about the placement, they will still be feeling very nervous about this first encounter and will remember every detail about it. Ideally either the practice supervisor and/or the practice assessor should be there on the student's first day, as this ensures that the student's learning journey with you starts off as you want it. Certainly one of them is needed when the initial interview is undertaken. As a practice supervisor or practice assessor you may be nervous meeting your student for the first time. If you have had contact before the first day that will help ease the nerves (or they could be greater if that initial contact did not go well), but the student will also be anxious about their first day.

How Students Feel When Starting a New Placement

MacDonald et al. (2016) describe the experience of 10 students preparing for, starting and leaving their practice placements. Some of the feelings and worries that students expressed are summarised as:

- Feeling:
  - Intimidated
  - Overwhelmed with the practical logistics of preparing for their placement (uniform, what to take with them)
- Worried about:
  - How staff will view them and whether they will be liked
  - The off-duty and how they will manage study and personal life around it
  - Walking on to the placement and joining handover
  - Understanding all the new terminology
  - Getting to know everyone, their names and roles
  - Finding their way around the placement

These worries and feelings are quite possibly similar to what it was like for you on your first day as a student or on your first day as a qualified nurse; this is worth remembering when students arrive on placement, as this can affect how they may come across at first before they have settled in.

ORIENTATION

One of the best ways to ensure that a student feels welcome to the practice placement is to orient them to the placement environment as soon as possible. Ideally, orientation should be a staged process during the first day to ensure that the student is provided with all the information they require and that they are given the opportunity to ask questions that may be relevant to them. The student's PAD will have an orientation checklist in it that will need to be signed off. It is a helpful guide for planning that first day.

Try to start the orientation by showing your student the essentials; where to put their bag/coat, and the location of staff lockers or changing rooms if relevant. If possible, arrange for this to take place within the first few minutes of them arriving in the placement. If you have got a student locker or locked cupboard available for valuables, then make sure the student knows how to access this. Knowing where to put your personal property and how to access these items throughout the day will put them at ease very early on, as it shows that you are interested in their welfare.

The next step in the orientation involves introducing your student to the other staff on shift that day. Let everyone know the student's name and the year of the programme they are on and how long their placement will be. It is a good idea to let the team know whether you are the student's practice supervisor or practice assessor, so they are clear what your role is in relation to the student. If the practice assessor and practice supervisor are not there for the student's first day, then telling staff and the student who they are is important. Everyone has a role to play in supporting students and will need to provide feedback to the practice supervisor and assessor on their own experiences of working with the student, so knowing who to go to is important. The use of a notice board identifying the staff linked to each student is really helpful, and was discussed in Chapter 3. If you can introduce the student during handover then you won't have to repeat the information throughout the day (although reminders as to who is who are helpful, as the student will be absorbing a huge amount of information on their first day).

An introduction does not have to be long or complex, something simple will do:

> 'Hi everyone, I'd like to introduce you to Jenny. She's a third-year student and she is on placement with us for 6 weeks. Today's her first day and just to let everyone know, I'm her practice assessor and John is her practice supervisor.'

A simple and friendly introduction will allow greetings to be swapped. You can encourage your colleagues to introduce themselves and explain what their role is. If your practice area routinely does a handover, encourage your student to join in and ensure your student is provided with the same materials as other staff.

The second part of orientation will be to ensure that the student is oriented to the placement area and that health and safety issues are addressed. This will be a requirement in the PAD and so will need to be signed off by the person undertaking the orientation. The types of information your student will need are shown in Box 5.1, which is taken from the Pan London Practice PAD 2.0 (Pan London Practice Learning Group, 2019a).

Lastly, it is important that the student is aware of how to contact the placement, who to contact, and is provided with their off-duty for the placement. All these areas can be addressed throughout the first day to ensure that the student receives a thorough orientation without feeling overwhelmed.

BOX 5.1 Orientation Checklist

	Placement area 1	
Name of placement area:		
Name of staff member:		
This should be undertaken by a member of staff in the placement area	Initial/Date **(Student)**	Initial/Date **(Staff signature)**
A general orientation to the health and social care placement setting has been undertaken		
The local fire procedures have been explained Tel..................		
The student has been shown the: ● Fire alarms ● Fire exits ● Fire extinguishers		
Resuscitation policy and procedures have been explained Tel:		
Resuscitation equipment has been shown and explained		
The student knows how to summon help in the event of an emergency		
The student is aware of where to find local policies ● Health and safety ● Incident reporting procedures ● Infection control ● Handling of messages and enquiries ● Other policies		
The student has been made aware of information governance requirements		
The shift times, meal times and reporting sick policies have been explained		
The student is aware of his/her professional role in practice		
Policy regarding safeguarding has been explained		
The student is aware of the policy and process of raising concerns		
Lone working policy has been explained (if applicable)		
Risk assessments/reasonable adjustments relating to disability/learning/pregnancy needs have been discussed (where disclosed)		
The student has been shown and given a demonstration of the moving and handling equipment used in the placement area		
The student has been shown and given a demonstration of the medical devices used in the placement area		

(Modified from Pan London Practice Learning Group, 2019a.)

> ! If your placement area has a student folder, try to include some of the orientation information in here. Phone numbers and key staff in the placement are very useful to include. On the first day you can ask them to read the information in the folder if it has not already been given to them before they start, and then ask any questions they may have.

THE INITIAL INTERVIEW

The initial interview is the first opportunity that you and your student will have to plan and discuss what is expected by you both on the placement. The NMC SSSA standard does not specify who will undertake the different elements of the practice assessment, but key statements indicate roles and responsibilities related to the student's time in practice, in particular:

> *Practice supervisors* 'support learning in line with their scope of practice to enable the student to meet their proficiencies and programme outcomes' and 'support and supervise students, providing feedback on their progress towards, and achievement of, proficiencies and skills' *(NMC, 2018b, p. 6).*

> *For practice assessors,* 'assessment decisions by practice assessors are informed by feedback sought and received from practice supervisors' and 'there are sufficient opportunities for the practice assessor to periodically observe the student across environments in order to inform decisions for assessment and progression' *(NMC, 2018b, p. 9).*

The university will have agreed with practice partners whether the practice supervisor or practice assessor should undertake the initial interview and this should be identified within the PAD or on guidance provided to practice supervisors and assessors by the university. The initial interview is important as it is a chance to discuss each other's expectations; it also marks the beginning of the student's assessment journey. For this reason, you may decide not to schedule the initial interview for the first day of placement, as your student will be taking in so much new information, they may be overwhelmed. If it can be scheduled later in the week, the student has an opportunity to get to know more about the placement and what learning opportunities the placement can offer. However, the initial interview should occur in the first week of the placement, so a lot will depend on when the practice supervisor and/or practice assessor have been scheduled to be on duty with the student during their first week.

Planning the Initial Interview

As said above, it is best practice to stage the initial interview in the first week of placement. If possible, try to decide the date and time of the initial interview during the student's first day of placement, so that you can both plan for the event. If you are both working the same off-duty, then scheduling the initial interview during a shift that you are both working in the first week should not be difficult.

When scheduling the initial interview try to allow at least 1 hour of protected time. This is not to say that the interview will always take 1 hour; however, by identifying this time you are creating a fixed period of time that can be planned for within the workload of others. You may want to consider planning the initial interview for a day in the first week when you know there is a good staff skill mix, or a day that is typically quieter than others. For example, a surgical placement may select the day when there is no elective surgery planned. This would allow the student and the practice supervisor/assessor to take an extended lunch together of 1 hour once everyone else has returned from their lunch break. This could be planned for in the off-duty; the other staff on duty that day can cover the lunch break without compromising patient care. Equally, a community placement may find the afternoons a better time for the initial interview if most home visits are undertaken in the morning.

It is important that both you and your student are prepared for the initial interview so that you can use the time constructively. Ensure that your student is aware they will need to ensure the following is available for the interview:

● Their PAD and their ongoing achievement record (OAR) from the previous placement if a paper version is used, or access to the student's e-PAD.
● Any supporting documents: for example, reasonable adjustments to be made.

In addition, make sure you are fully prepared yourself by reading through the professional values and proficiencies the student will need to achieve on their placement in advance of the initial interview. Also familiarity with the student's programme is invaluable as it ensures you have an understanding of what they have covered in their programme so far.

Staging the Initial Interview

The initial interview event will involve a mixture of discussion, recording information, and reading of materials. For this reason, it should take place in a location where there is an opportunity to sit comfortably at a table where both you and your student can write or access the PAD if on-line. If possible arrange to hold the interview in a quiet location away from the general hubbub of the clinical area, so that interruptions can be kept to a minimum.

Nurse's stations, clinic rooms, cars and cafeterias are usually the types of places to avoid for initial interviews. They are either not quiet, not comfortable, or not private. Ideally, you should be holding the initial interview in a meeting room, office, teaching room, etc; somewhere that a door can be closed, and noise kept out. If it is acceptable, put a sign on the door to stop interruptions. Just one hour of protected time at the beginning of a student's placement is worth its weight in gold for both of you.

Beginning the Interview

The initial interview is the first stage in the assessment process during the student's placement. It does not, however, need to be held in a formal style, in fact the more relaxed and informal this event the better for everyone involved. It is formal in the sense that the purpose of the initial interview is to develop an agreed contract of learning and assessment that can be followed and referred to during a student's placement. The initial interview is essential because it sets up an agreement of what learning opportunities the student requires to achieve the proficiencies in the PAD and how this will be supported. Without an initial interview, the student is essentially just working in your clinical area without any agreed direction. After the initial interview, the activities the student participates in will be contributing to their learning. Your assessment of their proficiency and ability to meet professional values will be part of an agreed plan for learning between the practice supervisor and the practice assessor and the student.

It's a good idea to have a checklist of issues that need to be covered at the initial interview so that you make the best use of time. At the very least, the following will need to be discussed:

- Prior practice experience before this placement
- Learning styles
- Any reasonable adjustments required
- Learning outcomes for the placement
- A plan of how learning experiences will be provided
- Expectations of competence
- Off-duty including confirmation of shift times to ensure regular contact with the practice supervisor and practice assessor
- Additional learning experiences or goals the student would like to achieve
- An agreement regarding expectations of feedback.

LEARNING STYLES

It is quite common to begin an initial interview with a student by asking them what they would like to learn. While the intention of this question is well meant, it rarely leads to a satisfactory answer, especially if it is a junior student. This request can leave the student floundering for what to say and how to proceed next. A far better way to commence an initial interview is to determine how your student prefers to learn, their learning style. This can provide some direction in planning their learning. There are many different approaches to categorising learning style; the learning styles suggested by Honey and Mumford (2006) in Box 5.2 tend to be the most popular and easiest for most people to relate to. During your initial interview it is very useful to determine what predominant learning style your student may have, as this can make planning of learning experiences far easier for both of you.

BOX 5.2 Honey and Mumford Learning Styles

Activists
Activists like to take direct action. They are enthusiastic and welcome new challenges and experiences. They are less interested in what has happened in the past or in putting things into a broader context. They are primarily interested in the here and now. They like to have a go, try things out and participate. They like to be the centre of attention.

Reflectors
Reflectors like to think about things in detail without taking any action. They take a thoughtful approach. They are good listeners and prefer to adopt a low profile. They are prepared to read and re-read and will welcome the opportunity to repeat a piece of learning.

Theorists
Theorists like to see how things fall into an overall pattern. They are logical and objective systems people who prefer a sequential approach to problems. They are analytical, pay great attention to detail and tend to be perfectionists.

Pragmatists
Pragmatists like to see how things work in practice. They enjoy experimenting with new ideas. They are practical, down to earth and like to solve problems. They appreciate the opportunity to try out what they have learned or are learning.

(From Honey and Mumford, 2006, pp. 19–20. With permission of Peter Honey Ltd.)

! Don't forget to work out your own learning style before asking the student about theirs. This way, you will be able to predict potential clashes in style and plan how to overcome any challenging situations.

Determining Learning Styles

The best way to determine your student's preferred learning style is for them to undertake a formal learning style questionnaire—for example, the 80-point questionnaire developed by Honey and Mumford (2006). However, from a practical point of view this will just not be possible during an initial interview. You can, however, get some indication of your student's learning style by asking just a few questions.

1. *On previous placements have you preferred to observe others demonstrating a task before undertaking the task yourself?* A yes answer may indicate a preference for a reflector or theorist style.
2. *On previous placements have you preferred to get 'stuck in' and undertake a task rather than observing others undertaking it first?* A yes answer may indicate a preference for an activist or pragmatist style.

3. *On previous placements have you tended to ask for explanations of treatment or care interactions before taking part in these activities?* A yes answer may indicate a preference for a reflector or theorist style.

4. *On previous placements have you tended to ask for explanations of treatment or care interactions after taking part in the treatment or care interactions?* A yes answer may indicate a preference for an activist or pragmatist style.

If it is their first placement, then asking them how they learnt best at school or college may provide an indication of their preferred learning style.

Determining your student's preferred learning style early in the initial interview is invaluable. Don't forget to share what this means with them. For example, if you think that they may be a theorist then share with them that you will try to point them to useful resources they can use to prepare for some of the patient treatments or care activities they will participate in as part of their learning experience. Also remember to share what your preferred learning style with the student is, as potential misunderstandings can be avoided if you are both clear about how you prefer to learn. For example, if you are an activist but your student is a theorist, there will be a clash of approaches to learning. As an activist you will view new learning opportunities as exciting and interesting and want to learn by doing. As a theorist the student will want to know more before engaging and may ask questions and ask to read the patient's notes or look up the procedure first, so that they have a clear picture and understanding of what they need to do and why, especially if it is something they have not done before. As an activist you may have felt that the student was reluctant to get involved, or found it difficult to relate to their need to ask lots of questions first. Understanding how they learn best can assist you in appreciating their approach to learning and supporting their specific learning style.

Developing Alternative Learning Styles

The fact that your student may be predisposed to one particular style of learning does not mean that you should not encourage them from using a range of learning techniques within their placement experiences. There will be many situations where it is valuable for a student to utilise different skills and approaches to learning in order to achieve their proficiencies. For example, in an emergency situation, thinking fast and accurately on your feet is an imperative. There is not always time to consider options. Conversely, when needing to look at tables, charts and assessment results from a number of sources, the ability to think about and consider the best possible course of action requires a more theorist or reflector approach. Learning to be a nurse will also mean learning how to use a range of different learning styles appropriate for the different situations you and your student will find yourselves in. There are some examples of where developing the ability to use different learning styles is valuable in Box 5.3.

BOX 5.3 Using Different Learning Styles

Why do I need to be an activist?

If your least preferred learning style is 'activist' then it is likely that you will not enjoy learning when it involves a new experience or where there are fresh problems to solve. This will create some problems for you in your nurse training as there will be times when action is required and you will need to 'think on your feet.' For example, emergency situations or rapid changes in a patient's clinical condition will require you to make fast and competent decisions as part of a team. This is not the time to spend time thinking through problems or deliberating over the best course of action. Crucially, a part of your learning will be to demonstrate that you can act and react under pressure.

Why do I need to be a reflector?

If your least preferred learning style is 'reflector' then it is likely that you will not enjoy learning experiences that involve observing problems or thinking through previous experiences. You will probably not enjoy investigating different types of research and ideas and may even feel like these activities are a waste of time. However, to demonstrate competence as a nurse you will need to be aware of best practice guidelines and take time to explore alternatives that support evidence-based practice. For example, new wound care techniques or drug therapies may require changes to your clinical practice.

Why do I need to be a theorist?

If your least preferred learning style is 'theorist' then it is likely that you will not enjoy spending time over decisions, or lengthy discussions over the best course of action. You may find attention to detail tedious, and become frustrated if you cannot get the answer straight away. However, such skills are vital for nurses. Whether it is a complex drug calculation or reading carefully through case notes and previous treatment plans, there will be a time when you will need to take the time to carefully think through problems before acting.

Why do I need to be a pragmatist?

If your least preferred learning style is 'pragmatist' then it is likely that you will not enjoy trying out new techniques or changing the way you do things. You may not be particularly interested in the consequences of actions or outcomes of events. However, 'pragmatic' skills are essential as these activities are strongly linked to evidence-based practice and being able to adapt and change patient care plans so that the best treatment options are delivered. This includes a range of activities, from monitoring fluid and electrolyte balance to re-evaluating a discharge plan.

(From Sharples, 2009, pp. 46–47. With permission from Learning Matters.)

It is important not only to try to develop learning experiences that support a student's learning style, but also to support the student by providing learning experiences that develop a range of styles. This is best done at the initial interview, where careful planning of potential learning experiences can be discussed and strengths and areas for development can be identified.

IDENTIFYING WHAT THE STUDENT NEEDS TO ACHIEVE ON THEIR PLACEMENT

Once you have gained some insight into your student's preferred learning style, the next stage of the initial interview is to take a very close look at the PAD to identify what needs to be achieved on the placement and if there are any elements in the PAD that may be problematic to achieve in your practice area. If the OAR is a separate document, it is important to look at this as well. We will start with this document first.

Reviewing the Ongoing Achievement Record

If the university your student is from has a separate OAR, then this is a good document to look at first, as it summarises the student's achievements on previous placements and should identify areas that the student needs to develop further. If the university uses a combined PAD and OAR then it is just one document (paper or electronic) to look at. These areas for development should be discussed with the student and become part of the plan for the types of learning experiences that they will require in your practice area. For example, if feedback from a previous placement has said that the student needs to improve their skills in identifying priorities and planning the work that needs to be achieved during a shift, then this will be an area that needs to be focussed on in addition to specific proficiencies. This will become an additional learning outcome the student will need to focus on during their placement. An action plan or agreement may be developed on how the student will achieve this during their placement with you.

Proficiencies

Depending on whether this is the first placement in the part/year of the programme or later in the year the choice of proficiencies will vary. If a first placement in the part/year, then you will be selecting from all the proficiencies. If it is a placement at partway through the part/year, then you will have a reduced number to choose from. Identifying what can be achieved on your placement is important so that you can identify what learning opportunities the student needs to be offered. If it is the final placement for the part, then all outstanding proficiencies will need to be achieved to enable the student to progress to the next part.

Previously Failed Proficiencies

When going through the PAD you may find that the student has failed one or more proficiencies or an episode of care/in-placement assessment and so these will be a priority for the student on this placement. You will need to identify with the student the learning opportunities they need in order to practice these proficiencies to enable them to be reassessed on them.

Episodes of Care/in-placement Assessments and Medicines Management

In addition to the proficiencies, there may be episodes of care or in-placement assessments where the student has to demonstrate a holistic approach to a patient/service user or group of patients/service users or they may be required to supervise and teach a student or other member of the team. The development of proficiency in medicines management will also be required, with the student demonstrating increasing proficiency for a wider group of people as they progress through their programme. Again, if it is the final placement for the part, then any episodes of care/in-placement assessments and medicines management assessments not yet completed will need to be achieved on this final placement if at all possible.

Sometimes it can be difficult to see how some of the proficiencies or additional in-placement assessments can be achieved in your particular practice area. If any of these prove problematic, then consideration of alternative approaches to achieving these will be needed, which we will look at in the next chapter.

IDENTIFYING LEARNING EXPERIENCES

The proficiencies and other assessments within the PAD that the student is required to undertake during the placement will largely determine the learning experience you should provide for them. For example, if the student has a proficiency related to drug calculations then you will be required to provide learning experiences where drug calculations may be undertaken, for example drug rounds, administration of insulin or calculating drugs being administered intravenously. From this point of view determining a learning plan/contract/agreement at the initial interview is a fairly straightforward affair. Discussing the learning experiences available and how these will be provided allows both you and your student to discuss expectations on both sides and troubleshoot foreseeable difficulties. This should include an honest discussion of any difficulties highlighted in the student's OAR. There will be a need to negotiate appropriate learning opportunities. For example, you might suggest to your student that they practise drug calculations on the midday drug round rather than the morning round, if this is a quieter time of day and allows more time for discussion and feedback. If you are community based then you may need to consider which patients or service users require medications to be given and arrange for the student to visit them or consider other learning opportunities that may be available to achieve this assessment requirement.

This is the time also to take note of your student's preferred learning style. If your student is a reflector, they may wish to observe you performing calculations and discuss the results before attempting drug calculations themselves. Alternatively, if your student is an activist, they may wish to perform drug calculations straight away and discuss these once they have calculated the result. In this case either approach to the learning experience has equal validity, and will ultimately allow you to assess their proficiency.

However, in practice whilst many routinely occurring learning opportunities can be planned for, many other learning opportunities will be opportunistic and as a consequence may not always suit theorists or reflectors. If your student leans to a reflector or theorist style of learning, then use some time during the initial interview to discuss ways as to how they can step forward and utilise these opportunistic learning experiences. The main point is that by establishing a learning plan at the initial interview both you and your student will be focused on the proficiencies they aim to achieve and a clear plan for how this can be achieved throughout the placement. Chapter 6 will explore how the proficiencies and other assessment requirements can be used to plan the learning experiences for students in more detail.

ADDITIONAL LEARNING OBJECTIVES

Apart from the proficiencies and other assessments within the PAD, it may be that your student has some personal learning objectives they would like to achieve during the placement. The initial interview is a great time to discuss these objectives. These may be related to a future career plan or a particular interest area they have or relate to an assignment they are undertaking, or topics covered in class. In the past there were certain practical skills that students were not allowed to undertake but the NMC Standards of Proficiency (2018d) now encompass a far wider range of skills, many of which were not standard before and seen as only appropriate for registered nurses or relevant only to specific fields. Appendix 1 lists some of these skills, which students from all four fields of practice are expected to achieve, although the level of proficiency will depend on their field of practice and exposure to each of the skills listed. The OAR may also indicate areas where the student has excelled, and you may both wish to set goals that will extend their proficiency in these areas further. This may relate to working with particular client groups or giving a succinct handover of a patient or service user which can be extended to handover of a larger group. Set objectives for these additional areas during the initial interview so that they can be planned for at the same time as the key learning objectives.

DISCLOSURE OF A DISABILITY

It will not be uncommon for a student to disclose that they have a disability. Unfortunately, some students prefer not to disclose disabilities at all for fear of discrimination. This often occurs after they have experienced a negative response by a practice supervisor or assessor in the past. Some students may not disclose a disability to you until they are some weeks into the placement, perhaps waiting until they have established trust before disclosing this information. Chapter 11 of this book explores how you can support students with disabilities or who have a specific learning need.

Having said this, the initial interview is a prime opportunity for a student to disclose whether they require any reasonable adjustments to be made. The need to check for this now appears on most orientation checklists. This provides you with an opportunity to raise the subject with each student, rather than hoping they will raise it themselves. You can simply ask if there are any reasonable adjustments or specific needs that they want to share with you. Remember, it is their right not to say anything and the initial interview should proceed on the understanding that if they choose not to disclose then you are not in a position to put any reasonable adjustments in place and cannot take these into account when planning learning opportunities.

If a student does choose to disclose a disability to you at the initial interview, then you should ask your student about the nature of the disability and how this may affect their learning experience. You can also ask for any supporting information that they may have been provided with by the university in terms of reasonable adjustments that may be required. You can use the information that the student provides to plan their learning experience and make adjustments to the learning plan as required.

> ! If a student does disclose a disability at the pre-visit or initial interview and you are unsure of how best to support the student, seek advice from the Link Lecturer at the university as soon as possible.

EXPECTATIONS OF STUDENT PROFICIENCY

It is virtually impossible to develop a learning plan without discussing and agreeing with your student what expectations you have of what achievement of a proficiency looks like. Remember that students are undertaking the placement not only for learning experiences to be provided, but also to determine their competence reflected through achievement of the professional values and proficiencies. Chapter 6 will explore further the types of evidence that are required for a student to demonstrate achievement of the required proficiencies and professional values. Whether you are a practice supervisor or practice assessor you must be confident about your expectations of what level of proficiency is expected for each of the proficiencies and what behaviours should be demonstrated in relation to the professional values from the outset. You must share and discuss these expectations with your student when developing each learning plan. It is very helpful if you not only document the learning plan in their assessment document, but also make a note of what you will be expecting in order to assess the outcome as achieved. Remember that your expectations of behaviours and proficiency should include equal measures of knowledge, skill and professionalism. It is worthwhile spelling out from the beginning exactly what these expectations are for each element to be assessed within the PAD and what you will be looking for in order to sign them off as having been achieved or to provide feedback to the practice assessor.

If you are vague or unclear about what is expected it can confuse the student. Being clear as to what is expected of them provides them with goals to aim towards. Your student should also be made aware that their assessment will be based on evidence from a wide variety of sources, and that practice supervisors and other registered health and social care professionals will contribute to the overall assessment of the student that the practice assessor will make.

After deciding on a learning plan and making expectations clear it is very important that you document all these considerations in the student's PAD. Not only does this provide the evidence of what has been discussed, it also provides a very clear benchmark of what should take place during the placement. It is likely that your student will work alongside many others during the placement and if expectations are well documented then the student will be able to show the learning plan developed at the initial interview as a guide for learning when you are not present. Documentary evidence of the learning plan developed at the initial interview will also provide the basis for feedback throughout the placement. Both you and your student will be able to refer to the agreement made at the initial interview as a basis on which to discuss progress and achievement of objectives. In essence it is not really any different from a plan of care for a patient or service user, which is used as a communication tool between everyone involved in their care and as a record of care planned and given.

! While the students in your clinical area may change, the learning experiences available to students will probably stay the same. Why not agree within your team the types of experiences suitable to students in each stage of their programme and the expectations of proficiency for each proficiency or assessment element? In this way students will be provided with a good range of experiences and are more likely to be assessed fairly by all practice assessors.

Planning the Off-duty

While the development of a learning plan and expectations are the focus of the initial interview, there are additional elements to this event which must not be forgotten. No matter how good your learning plan is, it will not be effective unless your student spends the majority of their placement working with their named practice supervisor(s) with regular days identified for the practice assessor to work with them. Both practice supervisors and assessor must make a commitment to ensuring that the student spends enough time with each of them to enable a fair and accurate assessment of their proficiency. In order to achieve this goal you should aim to provide the student with the same off-duty as yourself. If there are days or nights when this is not possible then arrange another named practice supervisor for the student, someone who can follow up on progress on your behalf and also provide clear and accurate feedback. This person will need to be briefed on the learning plan and expectations of competence also – so all the more reason to write this down at the initial interview.

It is crucial that you make time in the initial interview to clarify the off-duty with your student, and ascertain if there will be any difficulties for them following your work rota. If there are difficulties in terms of family or work commitments, then these must be highlighted. If there are any concerns this should be discussed with the university.

> ! It will be impossible to undertake a continual assessment of your student's progress unless you spend sufficient time together. Use the initial interview to plan the off-duty to maximise your opportunity to supervise and assess student competence.

SCHEDULING FEEDBACK

The completion of the initial interview will mark the beginning of the assessment phase during the student's clinical placement. For this reason it is very important to negotiate with your student a schedule of times for feedback during the placement experience. You should aim to discuss the frequency of feedback and what will be covered during feedback. Chapter 7 of this book will look specifically at feedback so we won't go into too much detail just now. However, it is important that you discuss what your student can expect from you in terms of feedback during the placement at the initial interview. If you are planning on providing informal feedback then the student should be prepared for this. In addition, you should also plan for formal feedback events, specifically the midpoint interview. If possible, try to agree on the date of the midpoint interview with your student at the end of the initial interview. It can then be a set event that you both plan for and prepare for in advance.

PERSONALITY CLASHES

Like all human relationships, clashes of personality between a student and a practice supervisor/assessor can occur. Personality clashes are less likely if you are prepared for the student and the placement gets off to a good start for both of you. The risk of personality clashes can also be reduced if there is clear and friendly communication between you and your student early in the placement, and the initial interview is the ideal time to cement a positive working relationship. Remember that your role in developing an effective student-supervisor/assessor relationship is to provide appropriate learning experiences and to undertake a fair and accurate assessment of the student's proficiency. You are required to be friendly toward your student but the relationship must remain a professional one to enable feedback to be effective.

UNDERSTANDING THE DOCUMENTATION

At the end of the initial interview you should clarify with your student how the documentation within the PAD will be completed. In Chapter 4 we identified the key elements of a PAD; however, changes can take place and you must make sure that you are familiar with the one being used for each placement. It is not uncommon for PADs to vary slightly between first-, second- and third-year students so don't assume they are all the same.

Access to the Practice Assessment Document

If the PAD is a paper document, then you should also ensure that your student is clear regarding when you will need to see the PAD after the initial interview. If you want it available daily so you can review learning outcomes, then make this clear. If your student is concerned regarding how to keep the document safe, then offer them a locked cupboard or room if you have not already done so. While these may seem small issues they can easily be the source of controversy and disharmony if not clarified from the outset. If the student has an e-PAD, access is much easier, depending on what has been agreed regarding access between practice partners and the university. For example, for some universities the agreement may be that the practice assessor has a log-in and can access the e-PAD at any time but practice supervisors can only access the e-PAD with the student present.

Contact Numbers

It is often useful to have a student's contact details, for example, phone number or email, so that you can contact them if needed during the placement. The student does not have to provide you with these as they are personal information so an explanation as to why this is useful should be provided. Discuss contact details with the student at the initial interview and clarify the situations that you will contact them under. This may include an unplanned change to the shift pattern or if you are concerned about unexplained non-attendance. You will need to make it clear that you will keep their details for the placement period only, and not disclose them to others.

! Contact details of students must be kept in a secure place and never disclosed to third parties. This information should be destroyed safely after completion of the placement. If a student does not wish to disclose their private contact details, then ensure you are aware how to contact them via the university or their university email.

MAKING THE MOST OF THE INITIAL INTERVIEW

The initial interview is your best opportunity to establish very clearly with the student what your role is (practice supervisor or practice assessor) during the placement. It is your chance to clarify exactly what they can expect from you in this role and to form a positive working relationship. If you leave the initial interview to chance you run the risk of conducting it in a rush or conducting it too late in the placement to be of benefit. To avoid this you will need to prepare for and schedule the initial interview as a distinct event during the student's first week of placement. You will also need the support of your colleagues to ensure the event is not interrupted. However, time spent at this stage will not be wasted, and can prevent potential problems from occurring later in the placement. The initial interview allows you and your student to clarify the nature of your relationship and set clear boundaries and expectations that will form the basis of all future placement decisions.

Action Points

- Try to schedule a student's initial interview into the planned off-duty for the first week. Ask your colleagues to cover your work so that the time can be ring-fenced.
- Undertake a review of learning styles and identify your own learning style as this will help you to understand similarities and differences in how you and your student approach learning.

Chapter 6

Planning Learning Opportunities

Chapter Outline

INTRODUCTION

The Nursing and Midwifery Council (NMC) *Standards of proficiency for registered nurses* (2018d) require student nurses regardless of the field of practice to achieve the same proficiencies. Whilst the proficiencies can be interpreted to reflect the people they are caring for, this can sometimes pose a challenge to the practice supervisor and practice assessor in planning the learning opportunities for the students they are supporting. The approach used by practice supervisors and assessors in planning the range of learning opportunities that a student needs to experience

A Nurse's Survival Guide to Supervising and Assessing. https://doi.org/10.1016/B978-0-7020-8147-7.00006-5

to enable them to meet the NMC proficiencies will vary depending on a number of factors. These include the type of placement, the types of experiences available and how they align with the proficiencies that need to be met. The experience of the practice supervisor and practice assessor in supporting students and understanding what the student needs to achieve will influence how successful the placement is for the student. A key skill is recognising unplanned learning opportunities as they arise and the ability to use the 'teachable moment'. This chapter explores the different types of proficiencies students are required to achieve. Examples of proficiencies and other assessments found within practice assessment documents will be looked at and broken down to show how this can help to identify what the student needs to demonstrate to achieve the assessment criteria. Approaches to enabling learning opportunities in different types of practice placements will be explored with consideration of how learning opportunities outside of the traditional placement can offer students the experiences they require to achieve their assessment requirements. This chapter starts by looking at why recognition of supernumerary status is so important in enabling students to access the range of learning opportunities they require.

SUPERNUMERARY STATUS

The NMC Standards set out expectations of student support in practice. This includes the requirement that they '*are allocated and can make use of supported learning time when in practice*' (NMC, 2018e, p. 14). Supported learning time, is time which will enable the student to learn and achieve their proficiencies with the support and facilitation they require. For pre-registration nursing students and direct entry nursing associates this includes being supernumerary '*in practice or work placed learning* and they *must be supported to learn without being counted as part of the staffing required for safe and effective care in that setting*' (NMC, 2018c, p. 18). Supernumerary status also applies to student nurse apprentices except when they are in their substantive work-based area. Nursing associate apprentices are required to have assured protected learning time. The level of supervision students require however will be dependent on their experience and level of proficiency. Whilst this should develop as they progress through the programme some placements may see an increased need for supervision until the students gain confidence and acquire further proficiency in the new area of practice. The decision about the level of supervision a student requires will be made by the practice supervisor and assessor. A word of caution though; a confident student is not necessarily a proficient one! It is therefore essential that each new student is supervised until the practice supervisor and assessor are able to make a decision on the level of supervision they will require during their time on placement.

IDENTIFYING LEARNING OPPORTUNITIES

A significant part of the practice supervisor's role is to facilitate student access to the learning opportunities they need. The practice assessment document/ongoing achievement record (PAD/OAR) will set out the proficiencies that need to be met and any additional assessment requirements that need to be met such as episodes of care/in-placement assessments, assessments on medication management and the assessment of specific clinical skills. As part of the initial interview the practice supervisor/assessor will have identified with the student what proficiencies need to be achieved and which are achievable in the placement. This will have been based on matching the proficiencies in the PAD to the different learning opportunities available in the placement to ensure that the ones selected are achievable. It is important to note that this is a joint decision. The NMC expects students to be empowered to take the lead on and responsibility for their own learning so encouraging the student to identify learning opportunities is important. However, the learning should relate to their proficiencies and this requires an understanding of what the proficiencies mean.

INTERPRETING PROFICIENCIES

Interpreting what a proficiency means can sometimes be challenging because they can incorporate a number of requirements especially in the more advanced proficiencies. However, it is essential that both practice assessors and supervisors are familiar enough with the language used in order to determine what learning opportunities the student needs to access to enable them to achieve the proficiency. The terms used within a proficiency are a guide to what needs to be assessed.

When translating what each proficiency means to you, it makes sense to start with the verbs used in each statement. The translation of the verbs must also relate to a clinical learning experience rather than a direct definition from a dictionary so that they reflect nursing practice. A model that is helpful in understanding how learning outcomes and proficiencies are developed and assist you in identify the learning that the student is required to demonstrate is Bloom's taxonomy of educational objectives developed by Bloom in 1956.

Bloom's Taxonomy of Educational Objectives

Bloom's taxonomy of educational objectives (Bloom et al 1956) is a model with three domains which are to structure learning objectives: the cognitive domain (knowledge and understanding), the psychomotor domain (skills) and the affective domain (values and beliefs).

The Cognitive Domain

The cognitive domain is the one most widely known and used by teachers, although the two other domains are clearly very applicable to nursing. Bloom used a hierarchy of nouns to create a hierarchy of thinking skills:

● knowledge
● comprehension

- application
- analysis
- synthesis
- evaluation.

This hierarchy was revised by Anderson et al. (2001) to turn the nouns Bloom used into verbs. This offers a more useful way of thinking as it reflects the actions of nurses in practice. The order of the hierarchy was also changed moving synthesis to the top of the hierarchy and renaming it as creating:

- remembering
- understanding
- applying
- analysing
- evaluating
- creating.

So, at the lower end is the ability to remember/recall facts and theory learnt, whereas at the top end is the ability to utilise a range of knowledge, facts and theories and create something new or to develop new meaning. Bloom's model can help you understand the type of knowledge and understanding a student is required to evidence in achieving a proficiency. Some examples of commonly used verbs found in PADs and their broad definitions are listed below. The list is not exhaustive, but it is a good place to start as it not only gives an idea of how students could make the most of the learning opportunity but also hints towards what sort of evidence you could ask the student to provide. The hierarchy starting with *remembering* and progressing through to the higher levels of cognitive skills of *evaluating* and *creating* can be related to the progress of the student through each part of the programme. You are therefore likely to find more of the verbs under remembering and understanding in a part 1 PAD and a greater use of the verbs under analysing, evaluating and creating in the parts 2 and 3 PADs.

Verbs Used in the Cognitive Domain

Remembering This includes recalling facts, definitions, etc. that have been previously taught or learnt. Verbs used are:

> *Describe:* Requires the student to tell you about the knowledge they have. This might relate to a specific assessment, an intervention, diagnosis or medication.
> *Select:* Requires the student to make an appropriate choice from a number of options.

Understanding This requires the student to demonstrate that they comprehend the facts, ideas or information they have gathered. Verbs used are:

> *Identify:* Requires the student to select from a number of options and be able to name the differences.

Recognise: Requires the student to differentiate between what was expected and what was not expected but where they may not have the language to define the differences or have the skills to respond, for example a student may recognise a person is vulnerable but not what they need to do.

Review: Requires a student to consider actions taken or options available and determine if a change is needed based on the information they have.

Applying This can include applying theory to practice, performing a skill or using a tool. Verbs used are:

Demonstrate: Requires the student to be able to perform a skill or apply knowledge and understanding of concepts and theories related to clinical practice.

Develop: Requires the student to create something in response to information gathered (a care plan) or to grow (professionally).

Use: Requires the student to select and apply an appropriate approach or tool in a given situation.

Analysing This can include selecting the relevant evidence needed to make a choice, a decision on the best approach and explain why. Verbs used are:

Apply: Requires the student to choose or select the right intervention based upon a sound evidence base and then put this into practice.

Respond: Requires the student to take an appropriate action or make the appropriate reaction in relation to an incident or event.

Evaluating To make a judgment using the evidence gathered or presented and select the best solution. Verbs used are:

Assess: Requires the student to measure, judge or weigh up the information gathered.

Evaluate: Requires the student to make a judgement or calculation on the importance or value of actions taken regarding a care task or information gathered.

Creating To create something new or useful. Verbs used are:

Develop: Requires the student to compile information to create something new, for example a plan of care.

Establish: Requires the student to start, create or develop new events or situations, for example therapeutic relationships.

Maintain: Requires the student to continue to perform to a given standard at all times once they have mastered the task, for example written documentation.

Process: Requires the student to gather, organise information to create something new such as a care plan.

! Keep a list and definitions of commonly used verbs within the PAD and develop a
folder for staff supporting students in your practice area with examples of how the
more difficult proficiencies could be achieved. This will help to ensure all staff in
the practice placement assess students according to the same criteria.

The Psychomotor Domain

Bloom did not fully develop the psychomotor and affective domains, but they
have been developed by a number of other authors. The one that fits well with
nursing is a version by Dave (1970) which describes the development of skilled
practice. The hierarchy has five levels from the initial learning of new skills to
skilled practice:

Imitation – learning skills by observing and then copying.
Manipulation – performing skills by memory or by following instructions.
Precision – skilled performance becomes more accurate.
Articulation – performing a series of skills together or adapting skills to meet
different circumstances.
Naturalisation – equates to performing skills without thinking about them
(like riding a bicycle).

It is not unusual to observe a junior student concentrating so hard on performing a new skill in practice that they forget the other behaviours that need
to be demonstrated alongside them and these tend to fall under the affective
domain.

The Affective Domain

The affective domain is particularly important in nursing as it about feelings,
emotions, attitudes, values and motivations. No matter how well a student performs a skill or how much they know about the theories related to the care that
they are giving, the approach used by the student is just as important. Again,
there are five levels, each progressing to increasing complexity. Many of these
will be innate in the student but they will also need to learn about and integrate
the professional values expected of them into their day-to-day behaviours.

Receiving phenomena: the awareness of feelings and emotions. This may be
demonstrated by the ability to listen attentively.
Responding to phenomena: this describes the active participation of the
student in a learning situation.
Valuing: this is the ability to see the worth of something and be able to express
the values involved.
Organisation: the ability to prioritise one value over another.
Characterisation: the ability to internalise values such that they become part
of who you are; the professional compassionate nurse.

Using the Domains to Help Structure Questions

The terms used in the three domains are useful to structure questions you may use with a student or to assist you in assessing a student. For example, if asking a first-year student questions you might ask them to *identify, select* or *list* but for a final placement student you might ask them to *evaluate* or *assess* a situation or their performance.

When reviewing a student's performance in a clinical skill (psychomotor skills) you would not expect a new student to be fluent in their performance (=naturalisation); instead they would need to observe and copy or be guided through each step by you.

The professional values are closely linked with the affective domain and a student may exhibit values across these domains moving to characterisation as they learn about and become socialised into the professional values expected of a nurse.

Applying the Domains to a Proficiency

To help with understanding how the domains apply in nursing let's see how the three domains can be applied to medicines management.

A junior student might be able to list some common medications, dispense a tablet and demonstrate interest in listening to their supervisor explain about the side effects. A senior student will undertake an assessment of a person in their care who is in severe pain or distress and then select the most appropriate medication to be given based on the evidence collected and administer it skilfully via the most effective route whilst demonstrating a non-judgemental professional attitude, responding with a caring and person-centred approach.

Bearing in mind how these three domains influence a proficiency, the ability to understand whether a proficiency is focusing on one domain or all three is important in determining what evidence will be required by the student to demonstrate that they have achieved it. The next step in the process therefore is to understand in more detail what the proficiency is actually requiring the student to do and may involve interpreting some of the language related to the proficiency statement.

Breaking a Proficiency Down

Sometimes breaking down the proficiency into smaller sections can help it become more meaningful and measurable. If you are unsure what a proficiency is asking the student to do, use the following process to break the proficiency down.

Step 1 – Identify and understand the relevant verb used in the proficiency. This is the key indicator as to what the student has to do.
Step 2 – Decide if the proficiency needs breaking down so that it is manageable.
Step 3 – Look for any hints of the types of learning opportunities in the statement that would enable the student to achieve the proficiency to enable you to identify the learning opportunities the student should engage with.
Step 4 – Decide what evidence will demonstrate proof of learning.

For steps 3 and 4 it is important to bear in mind the stage of the programme that a student is at as not all learning opportunities may be appropriate for a student on their first placement and the level of evidence will be less for a first year than for a final year student.

For example, the following is a long proficiency statement:

Accurately processes all information gathered during the assessment process to identify needs for fundamental nursing care and develop and document person-centred care plans.

Pan London Practice Learning Group (2019a)

If you break this down it becomes easier to identify what the student needs to do by using each of the steps above.

Step 1 – the verbs are *gathered* and *processes, identify* and *develop* and *document.* So a lot of different actions are required from the student.

Step 2 – this is a lengthy proficiency with a number of elements; if you break it down into its different parts it becomes clearer as to what is being asked:

a. Undertake an assessment of a patient/service user which includes all the information required to make a complete assessment. This may be a full admission assessment or completion of one or more of a range of different risk assessment tools depending on the student's stage in their programme and the reason why a patient/service user has been admitted.

b. Identify the needs of the patient/service user from the data gathered.

c. Develop a care plan to meet the individual's needs (person-centred).

d. Document (or record) the care plan as per local policy.

Step 3 – this proficiency clearly indicates what learning opportunities the student needs to access to enable them to achieve the requirements detailed in the statement. An ideal situation would be an admission assessment. It does not need to be for a complex care scenario as the focus is on fundamental nursing care needs. So, if a simple admission assessment is not easily available, the use of one or more assessment tools to identify a person's fundamental care needs such as a nutritional assessment or pain assessment, or use of risk assessment tools for falls or pressures sores could be undertaken and a care plan developed or adjusted to reflect the outcomes of the assessment tools used.

Step 4 – the evidence would be the completed care plan related to the assessment approach that was undertaken. However, note the word 'accurately' so the data gathered must be accurate as must the elements within the care plan. A discussion with the student's practice supervisor/assessor will also be required on the processes they used and whether the care plan met all the person's needs and was person-centred.

Once the proficiencies have been identified that can be achieved on the placement then the next step is agreeing how the student will access the learning opportunities they need and what evidence they will be required to provide to demonstrate achievement of the proficiency.

AGREEING THE EVIDENCE

Evidence is what the student will do/provide to demonstrate achievement of a proficiency, in other words, proof that learning has taken place. This evidence should be directly related to the proficiency, be applied to the learning opportunities available and the student must know what is expected of them right from the beginning. If you have been able to understand and communicate the meaning of the proficiency clearly then the evidence should follow easily. The evidence the student produces should be tangible and directly observed or reported back by the student during their placement. Depending on the type of proficiency the evidence may be quantifiable, for example, accurate documentation of a specific number of care plans. Evidencing softer skills can be more challenging and often requires a discussion. For example:

● Is aware of own unconscious bias in communication encounters (e.g. equality and diversity).

The evidence for this skill may require the student to discuss with you what is meant by unconscious bias and provide examples that have been explored at university. They may then provide an example of where they were communicating with a patient/service user or member of staff and became aware of personal biases and how they adapted their communication style to communicate effectively without bias.

Alternative Forms of Evidence

Sometimes proficiencies which are difficult to achieve in the placement cannot be delayed until the next placement. If the student is on the last placement for that part of their programme, then the PAD must be fully completed in order for the student to progress to the next part of the programme or qualify. In these situations considering more creative approaches as to how the student might demonstrate achievement of the proficiency or skill is required. Options are:

● a reflective discussion
● presentation of a resource that meets the proficiency
● participation in a simulated activity
● a discussion regarding the use of a specific assessment tool and the evidence base supporting it.

Some skills may be difficult for certain fields of practice to achieve outside of their own field and it is possible that the university has a plan in place to enable the student to achieve certain proficiencies through simulation at the university. If unsure check this out with the Link Lecturer.

Proficiencies that are Challenging to Achieve

There will always be some types of care activities which preclude the involvement of students to a greater or lesser degree. For example, some women may refuse certain care activities to be delivered by a male student nurse, a service user being visited by a community mental health nurse may not wish a student to be present at their meeting or parents may not wish a student to undertake venepuncture on their child. The NMC states that universities and practice partners must:

> *ensure people have the opportunity to give and if required, withdraw their informed consent to students being involved in their care.*

NMC (2018b, p. 6)

It is important that the reason why this request may be made by a patient or service user is explained. The student needs to understand and appreciate the patient or service user's perspective and also that this is not about them as a person. In these situations alternative activities can be explored which allows the equivalent learning to take place. Possible options are:

● accessing the simulation centre to practice female catheterisation or venepuncture on a mannequin
● reviewing a video of a service user's experience of mental illness – charity websites such as the Mental Health Foundation and Mind have videos and podcasts a student can review and then discuss with their practice supervisor or assessor.

As discussed in the last chapter, at one time universities would provide a list of clinical skills that students could not undertake in practice; these were often more advanced skills, but this no longer applies unless the organisation you work at has a policy which only permits registered nurses or other healthcare professionals to perform them. With the move to the 2018 NMC Standards healthcare organisations have reviewed many of these policies to enable students to practice these skills under the supervision of an appropriate healthcare professional. Appendix 1 at the end of the book lists the more advanced skills now required of all students regardless of field. Some of these skills may be ones that practice supervisors or assessors do not feel competent to teach to the student. In these situations it is worth considering who else may have these skills. Often this may be other healthcare professionals or staff such as doctors, physiotherapists or clinical nurse specialists (CNS).

DOCUMENTING THE LEARNING PLAN

An agreed plan should then be documented in the PAD identifying the proficiencies that have been selected, an agreement on how they will be achieved, and the evidence needed to demonstrate that the proficiencies have been achieved.

For example using the proficiency above, the following may be written in the learning plan:

Jenna will observe two admissions during her first week and then undertake an admission assessment and produce a completed care plan meeting the care needs of the person by her mid-point assessment.

This is known as a SMART objective and makes it very clear what is expected as shown below. The words in bold describe the activity and time scales.

Specific – it is very clear what activities Jenna must engage with and what type of learning opportunities are needed to do this (**admission assessments**).
Measureable – observe two admissions and undertake one admission. Produce a completed care plan.
Achievable – it appears achievable and is appropriate unless this is her very first placement and requires Jenna to be on duty when admissions occur.
Relevant – completion of admission assessments would relate to proficiencies in the PAD.
Time scaled – clear target dates are set; observe two admissions during her **first week** and then undertake an admission assessment and produce a completed care plan meeting the care needs of the person **by her mid-point assessment.**

It is an NMC requirement that students are clear about the process for assessing a proficiency or skill and the type of evidence that will be used to assess them. By clearly documenting what has been agreed the student is fully informed of what is expected and can share this with other practice supervisors and their practice assessor to ensure that the action plan is implemented. Without an agreed plan the student's learning may occur by accident rather than as planned and at the end of the placement you may find that very little has been achieved. This places the student in a difficult position as completion of all elements in the PAD is a requirement for progression to the next part of the programme. It is little wonder that students become obsessed with having their PAD completed.

Generally learning plans developed at the start of a placement tend not to use SMART objectives and are more general; however detailed learning plans provide many benefits as discussed above. SMART objectives are most commonly used at the mid-point interview where areas for improvement are identified or specific proficiencies or skills must be achieved by the end of the placement or in action plans where concerns have been raised regarding a student's performance. This will be looked at in Chapter 8.

MEDICINES MANAGEMENT AND PREPARATION FOR PRESCRIBING

A significant change with the 2018 NMC Standards for nursing was that they would prepare students to be ready to undertake a prescribing qualification at the point of registration with the NMC at the end of their programme. This more rapid progression has been facilitated by the NMC by replacing their *Standards of proficiency for nurse and midwife prescribers* with *A Competency Framework for all Prescribers* (Royal Pharmaceutical Society, 2016) and a number of professional guidance documents developed with the Royal Pharmaceutical Society. These have replaced their *Standards for medicines management* which restricted what students were permitted to do in relation to medicines management.

It should be noted that whilst a student should be ready to undertake a pre-scribing programme at the point of registration, in their first year they could only undertake a community practitioner nurse prescribing course (commonly called the V100 or V150) as they must be qualified and on the NMC regis-ter for a minimum of one year before undertaking the independent or supple-mentary prescriber programme (V300 course). The V300 has slightly different rules around practice supervisors and assessors. Nurses undertaking the V300 will have a practice assessor who is an experienced prescriber and a registered healthcare professional; the practice assessor does not need to be a registered nurse. In exceptional circumstances the same person can act as a practice super-visor and assessor as it is recognised that there may be difficulties finding two different people with the required experience and qualifications to undertake the two roles.

There are a number of proficiencies and clinical skills in the NMC *Standards of proficiency for registered nurses* related to anatomy, physiology, pharmacol-ogy, prescribing, medication management and administration that will ensure that the nurse is prepared with the knowledge and skills they will need to become prescribers. This will require practice supervisors and assessors to support stu-dents to achieve a more extended set of skills than was previously required when the focus was more on safe administration of medicines. Different countries have taken different approaches to incorporating the proficiencies and skills within their PADs related to medicines management with some using an in-placement assessment or episode of care which incorporates many of the skills and proficiencies and other countries requiring each proficiency and skill to be assessed separately.

Skills related to medicines management will start from year one, therefore requiring first-year students to be provided with opportunities to participate in administration of medicines. This can commence with the administration of medicines to a small number of patients or service users in the first part of the programme progressing to administration to a small group or caseload in the final year/part of the programme.

Nursing Associates

Nursing associates are also required to meet a number of proficiencies related to medicines management, many of which are similar to those for nurses but there is no requirement for them to be prescribing ready. They will need to be assessed on their proficiency in administering medicines to small groups of patients and service users.

EPISODES OF CARE OR IN-PLACEMENT ASSESSMENTS

Most universities include episodes of care or in-placement assessments within the PAD. These are holistic assessments which incorporate a number of proficiencies. They require selection of an individual or group of people who require a range of care activities and require the student to apply the achievement of the different proficiencies. This form of assessment needs forward planning and careful reading of the proficiencies and skills that the student is required to achieve to ensure that they meet the requirements of the assessment. A reflection may also need to be completed by the student and will form part of the evidence required.

INVOLVING OTHER HEALTH AND SOCIAL CARE PROFESSIONALS

The NMC Standards for student supervision and assessment (SSSA) Standards (NMC, 2018b) define practice supervisors as *'any NMC registered nurses, midwives, nursing associates, and other registered health and social care professionals'* (p. 6). Each of these professions can provide valuable learning opportunities for students enabling them to understand their roles and responsibilities and how their scope of practice differs from that of a nurse. In addition, planning opportunities for students to spend time with other healthcare professionals can be useful when the nominated practice supervisor or practice assessor is not scheduled to be on duty with the student. Planning and agreeing this time with the people identified is important especially in large organisations which have a lot of students to ensure they are not overwhelmed with requests. This may require the lead for practice in the organisation to liaise with the different professional groups and departments to agree a process for students to spend time with them. They will also need to be prepared to supervise student nurses and nursing associates. Examples of proficiencies and skills that can be learnt by spending time with other healthcare professionals are:

- chest auscultation from physiotherapists and doctors
- venepuncture and blood sampling from doctors or phlebotomists (note phlebotomists are not registered healthcare professionals)
- play therapy from a play therapist
- alternative communication techniques from a speech and language therapist
- therapeutic interventions such as motivational interviewing, solution focused therapies and positive behaviour support approaches from occupational therapists.

The Role of Healthcare Assistants in Student Learning

It is important not to forget that non-registered healthcare colleagues such as healthcare assistants (HCAs) also have a range of skills, knowledge and experience that students can learn about and are a valuable resource for students although they are not always appreciated by them (Elcock, 2020). Students can feel that they are being 'fobbed' off by their practice supervisor when allocated to work with an HCA, so time spent explaining the value to them is important. The majority of hands-on care activities in many settings are delivered by HCAs (Willis, 2015) and all students need to practice and learn these fundamental skills. Many HCAs also have an extended skill set including venepuncture, phlebotomy and 12-lead ECGs, and have been trained in specific interventions such as de-escalation and the management of violence and aggression. Working alongside HCAs therefore can provide opportunities for students to learn these skills from them. The practice supervisor or assessor can then discuss the evidence base underpinning these skills and interventions with the student to link theory with practice.

Clinical Nurse Specialists

CNSs offer a wide range of learning opportunities for students that may not be easily available in their placement or to enable a student to develop a wider understanding of an aspect of practice that they have seen on their placement. For example, a child field student could spend time with a CNS for diabetes who is visiting adults with diabetes to develop a greater understanding of the long-term impact of diabetes in children if their diabetes is not well controlled. A CNS as a practice supervisor can sign off a number of proficiencies, both those specific to their speciality and the wider skills they use around health promotion/education and teaching skills. They will also use a wide range of the communication and relationship management skills listed in Annexe A in the NMC *Standards of proficiency for registered nurses* (2018d) which can be found in the student's PAD.

Planning Time with Other Healthcare Professionals

If it is possible, agree with other health and social professionals a fortnightly or monthly time slot when students could meet with them to find out about their role. This would be fixed in time and place and they would not be overwhelmed by many calls from students and you would be able to prearrange for the student to attend. Ask the student to prepare for their time with them by considering what they want to know and learn about and to identify specific proficiencies and skills that might be achieved (junior students may require some help). The student will benefit from having a focused approach to the learning event, and the staff member they work with will be better prepared to talk about specific aspects of their role and involve the student with the care they deliver where it is appropriate.

Recording the Learning

There should be sections in the PAD where other health and social care professionals can provide feedback to the student. If they do this they should also record their details on the record of practice supervisors within the PAD. The student should also reflect on their experiences within their PAD, identifying what they learnt and how this learning can be used in the future. If appropriate, they should also include any areas for further development.

SUPERVISION AND ASSESSMENT IN DIFFERENT TYPES OF PLACEMENT AREAS

Individual clinical areas will bring unique challenges and different opportunities to the approaches used for supervision and assessment and to the learning experience available for students. These are generated by the nature of the service delivered. This could be the different types of health problems of the patients/service users, the health status of the patient/service user group or the very specialised nursing care delivered. Commonly heard by students is '*you can learn that on your next ward placement*' or '*you'll do plenty of that when you're in the community*'. Whilst this may be true, creative thinking can enable students to access a wider range of learning opportunities than a particular placement first appears to offer. The NMC requires all students to be supervised when in practice but that does not always have to be the designated practice supervisor, although the practice supervisor or practice assessor must have oversight of the student's learning within that placement. This allows students to undertake periods of time outside of their main placement (insight, spoke or enrichment opportunity) to widen their experience and learning opportunities. Key is that these experiences should be relevant to their programme and contribute to the proficiencies they need to develop. The NMC SSSA Standards state that universities along with their practice partners must ensure that:

> *students have opportunities to learn from a range of relevant people in practice learning environments, including service users, registered and non-registered individuals, and other students as appropriate.*
>
> NMC SSSA Standards (2018b, p. 5)

However, in doing so this must not compromise public safety.

Community Placements

Community services provide a very different type of learning experience for students. Unfortunately, these placements are at a premium, so for some fields the student may only get one placement in the community. This means that practice supervisors and assessors can be supporting students at any point on their programme from their very first placement to their very last placement. The NMC SSSA standards have opened up greater opportunities in the way that students are supported in practice. Now students can now spend time with a number of different practice supervisors with regular contact during the placement with the designated practice assessor. This is a significant change from the previous mentorship system where the student would often spend the majority of their placement with one mentor.

If it is a small GP practice, then the student may spend the majority of their time with the practice nurse. However, students should be helped to undertake a number of outreach placements with services that link with the GP practice to broaden their understanding of how different community services are integrated. If it is district nursing or health visiting team, community learning disability services or school nurses, then junior students are likely to accompany their practice supervisor throughout their placement. This means that they will often be working alongside their supervisor throughout their time on placement, again with some time planned to be with the practice assessor. This is a very different experience to being on a busy ward where a student may often have periods where they are less closely supervised or supervised at a distance. This closer working relationship in community services can be stressful for both the student and the practice supervisor/assessor. For the student they may feel as if they are constantly under observation and for the practice supervisor/assessor they may feel that there is pressure to be teaching all the time. For both, these feelings and perceptions may increase if the student is underperforming as it causes additional pressure for both.

Afternoons can sometimes be a challenge in community placements. This is often when the practice supervisor/assessor may be office-based, writing up notes and catching up on administration and where office space to include students can be a challenge. Out-reach placements are valuable at this time and offer the student a greater breadth of learning experiences, and in particular, opportunities for out of field experiences. Some practical tips to help support students successfully and manage the challenges of working in community settings are:

- Be honest about needing reflective (quiet) time to consider the patient/service user you have just seen or plan for the next one you will see and agree times when discussions will take place on the care activities and interactions that have taken place.
- Provide a timetable for each week indicating the established meetings the student must attend, for example referral meetings, case conferences, student drop-ins, clinics and when home visits will take place, along with dates and times for the initial, midpoint and final interview.
- For senior students allocate two to three patients whom they will get to know and learn how care is provided for these patients across the length of the placement – this way the student is not overwhelmed by unfamiliar people whom they may only see once or twice.

- Consider outreach opportunities with other services in the community such as spending a day with:
  - a GP
  - GP practice nurse
  - dieticians
  - community based CNS – diabetes, enuresis
  - nurse consultants
  - community midwives
  - Macmillan nurses
  - homeless centres
  - sexual health clinics
  - drug and alcohol services
  - pharmacist
  - counsellor
  - podiatrist
  - other community-based services run by charities or social services.
- Ask the student to develop a resource that might be used by other students or for patients/service users they have met who might benefit from guides or create a poster for the GP practice or clinic.
- If a number of students are based in the community setting at the same time then the Collaborative Learning in Practice (CLiP) model could also be considered (Williamson et al., 2020) with senior students working with junior students.

Unsupervised Visits in the Community

One dilemma faced by staff in community settings is whether they should let students undertake home visits by themselves. The NMC is very clear that any nurse or midwife who delegates duties to a junior member of staff, including students, remains accountable for the decision to delegate. It is advisable to double check if the university has a lone working policy specifically relating to students to guide you in making the decision to delegate unsupervised duties, but with final year students this may be especially appropriate. General guidance would be that if visiting people in their own homes they should be people that they have visited before and have previously delivered the care required under supervision. The person being visited should consent to the student visiting them. The student is aware of the actions to take should an emergency take place. Mobile phones now offer almost instant help should a student have any queries or concerns whilst making a home visit alone. At the end of the visits the student must have an opportunity to debrief/reflect with their practice supervisor.

Inpatient Placements

Most inpatient settings tend to have a greater capacity for students compared to community settings. Some inpatient wards could have an allocation of students across all three parts of the programme. This may vary in specialist wards/

departments where only final year students may have placements. Listed below are some practical strategies to help manage the learning experience on an inpatient ward.

- Allocate two to three patients/service users to each student whom they will get to know and learn how care is provided to meet their needs.
- Agree one or two projects that the students can work on together during their placement which they can have allocated time off the ward to research and prepare and present at an agreed handover.
- Encourage students to meet other professionals in the team or other services together as discussed above.
- Encourage students to attend drop-in or support surgeries if run by the university or practice leads in the organisation.
- Consider using the CLiP model (see Chapter 1) where you have large numbers of students allocated.

For some of these practical solutions you will notice there are similarities between the community and inpatient settings. This is because the challenges faced are often the same; the only difference is the setting in which it takes place.

Hub and Spoke Placements

Many universities are now using hub and spoke placements (also called outreach or insight placements) to maximise placement capacity and provide students with a greater breadth of experience. A hub and spoke placement is usually arranged by the university in partnership with practice partners. The student will gain the majority of their placement learning in one area (the hub or base placement) but will undertake one or more shorter placements in areas that relate to their hub placement. The hub placement may span a whole year but is more usually 6 or more weeks in length. The spokes may occur as a block of time or may be one day a week away from the hub. Examples of hub and spoke placements are:

- Hub – surgical placement. Spokes – operating department, recovery, endoscopy
- Hub – elderly care ward. Spokes – day centre, nursing home, community
- Hub – hospice. Spokes – Macmillan nurse, pain clinic
- Hub – community mental health team. Spokes – Crisis teams, a mental health charity (e.g. MIND), Improving Access to Psychological Therapies
- Hub – Learning Disabilities (LD), Child and Adolescent Mental Health Services (CAMHS). Spokes – community LD team, special schools.

Planning learning opportunities needs to be more organised to ensure that they are timed appropriately, and the PAD needs to be kept up to date to allow effective communication with practice supervisors as the student moves across all the placement areas.

OPPORTUNISTIC LEARNING AND TEACHABLE MOMENTS

As well as planned learning opportunities based on the proficiencies the student needs to achieve, practice provides a multitude of situations or events that offer opportunistic learning to take place. This type of learning cannot be planned and needs to be recognised by the practice supervisor or assessor and utilised as and when it happens. Opportunistic learning may be used to re-direct the plans for the student that day or be turned into a 'teachable moment'.

Opportunistic Learning

Opportunistic learning is where something arises in the practice setting that was not foreseen but offers a valuable learning opportunity for the student. Some students are very good at picking up on these and asking to be involved but some may need to have them identified for them. Examples of opportunistic learning events are:

- emergency admission of a patient/service user who is acutely unwell
- a person with mental health problems presenting in crisis
- a sudden deterioration in someone requiring rapid medical or nursing interventions
- a cardiac arrest
- a person who needs to be sent for an emergency investigation (e.g. a CT scan, x-ray, ultrasound etc.)
- a person with diabetes who is exhibiting signs of hypoglycaemia
- a child exhibiting sudden respiratory distress

Each of these events offer valuable learning opportunities for students from any field and inviting them to join you or the staff involved in situations like this is essential if they are to learn how to respond to unplanned events in practice. Often students can be left out of events like this and asked to continue with the more routine care activities. However, the point of supernumerary status for students is that it allows students to be able to access the learning opportunities they need. Where sudden events occur it can be difficult to plan what the student should do and will depend on their experience. For junior students asking them to observe and note how the multidisciplinary team communicate with each other and with the patient/service user may be appropriate. For more experienced students they may record any drugs administered or be asked to assist in activities such as drawing up drugs, running drips through or sitting with the parents if the situation involves a child or baby.

What is essential is that where the event that takes place is an emergency that there is an opportunity to discuss what took place with the student afterwards. This allows the student to ask questions about anything they did not understand and for the practice supervisor to check the student's understanding of what took place and why.

Teachable Moments

'Teachable moments' or 'T-moments' are terms that can also include opportunistic learning. They are valuable as they occur in real time and are often when a student may be most receptive to learning. They do not have to be related to sudden unforeseen events but may arise when a practice supervisor is with a student and a learning opportunity becomes suddenly apparent. Examples of teachable moments are described below.

● A student tells you they have washed patients all week and wants to do something different.

Your response might be to select one of the patients they washed and ask the student to explain what information they gained about the patient whilst washing them. They may say nothing much. This then becomes a T-moment where you could discuss what they observed about the patient during the wash. Ask the student what they saw that might tell them about the patient's health status, for example nutrition and hydration status, potential for infection, their circulatory status, the condition of their skin and potential for pressure ulcers, how easily or not the patient was able to move in bed and what that might indicate. All of this information can be gathered by a student whilst assisting a patient with meeting their hygiene needs or providing a bed bath. They should also be able to comment on the patient's mental status and whether there are any concerns that need to be explored further. Obviously, asking these questions should be done in a supportive way that helps the student appreciate how a good knowledge base and understanding is required to pick up on all the cues that giving a bed bath can provide. Equally there could be a discussion on the mental health benefits of the protected time that a bed bath gives for talking with a patient and what additional information can be elicited during this time.

● You are working with a student and ask him to undertake the admission of a young man, Robert, who is autistic. Robert has had several previous admissions with you so you know him well. The student tells you they have never met anyone with autism before and is clearly nervous about undertaking the admission assessment.

Your response might be to discuss Robert's background with the student and explain what autism is. You then undertake the admission yourself and ask the student to observe the communication skills you use when talking with Robert. Afterwards you discuss how and why your communication style was different with Robert than it might be with someone who is not autistic.

T-moments occur throughout everyday practice; the skill is in identifying them and then using them. They may occur when delivering care but can occur at handover when you notice a student looking confused when a particular service user or patient is being discussed. Taking time to pause and clarify and explain terms being used can be really helpful to students especially when they are in a very new environment where the language everyone uses appears incomprehensible to them.

Some other examples of T-moments described by Reynolds et al. (2020) are using commonly used assessment tools as the focus for learning, asking the student to lead on an activity rather than doing it yourself, encouraging students to talk with patients on a given topic (e.g. impact of their illness on their life) or encouraging students to think out loud when undertaking a care activity, explaining their understanding of what they are doing and why. The latter example also works the other way round. As an expert practitioner what is very obvious to you will not be to a student.

Bite-sized Teaching

Health Education England (HEE) advocates the use of bite-sized teaching sessions in practice as a valuable, high impact learning experience. These are 10-minute teaching sessions focussed on the needs of the practice area and delivered to the whole multidisciplinary team and do not require PowerPoint presentations. The example given by HEE is a 10-minute session on a physical health topic delivered once a week by a junior doctor on a mental health unit at handover (see https://www.hee.nhs.uk/our-work/mental-health/bitesized-teaching). This approach could also be used by nurses for students in their area by developing one-page cue cards on a range of common conditions seen in the placement.

MANAGING AN OVERLAP OF STUDENTS ON PLACEMENT

At times, due to the nature and timing of placements across three years of a programme and multiple universities sending students to the same organisation there could be an overlap of students in your placement. This can add to the number of people around; in some cases there could be more staff and students than patients! This may even result in a sense of competition amongst students for the best learning opportunities. It can also mean that some staff may not have a break from supporting students before the next one arrives. Preparation and planning for learning in these circumstances is essential and there are some things you can do to manage the crossover successfully. Using senior students who have been on the placement for a while (established) can help them to learn the supervisor and teaching skills they need to develop as part of their proficiencies.

- Ask one of the senior established students to orientate and induct the new student to the clinical area, the unit/hospital and staff (this will need oversight by the practice assessor).
- Ask the established student and new student to work together looking at a specific clinical issue encountered in that placement area, jointly prepare a presentation on the topic and then present it to the team at an agreed handover.

- Ask the established student to prepare detailed handover notes of the current patients, introduce and handover all the patients to the new student.
- Arrange for the new student to meet other professionals in the team during the crossover period.
- Consider spoke placements where some of the students can go for short periods, for example theatres during a surgical placement, and rotate through to reduce the overall number on the placement at any one time.
- Have a timetable of activities mapped out for the new student during the crossover.
- Have the off-duty completed for the crossover period in advance so that you can arrange for the students to be on shifts with their practice supervisor yet not all on the same shift at the same time.

! Ask the students already on placement with you to be involved in orientating new students providing an opportunity to assess the student's organisation, planning, communication, leadership and team working skills.

Planning learning opportunities may at first seem to require a lot of work. However this will become easier as you become familiar with the PADs and the proficiencies and skills the students need to achieve. Good preparation will also save a lot of time later in the student's placement as it ensures that proficiencies are achieved across the placement rather than playing catch-up at the end.

Action Points

1. Work with colleagues to agree what proficiencies can be achieved in your placement area and the learning opportunities appropriate for students at each stage of their programme.
2. For each proficiency agree what types of evidence would be appropriate for students at each stage of their programme.
3. Draw up a list of additional learning opportunities relevant to your area that are available with other health and social care professionals or in other departments or sites.
4. Ask your Link Lecturer if the university has a guide for practice supervisors and practice assessors that will assist you with identifying learning opportunities.
5. Review the NMC's practice environment case studies which provide examples of how students can achieve their proficiencies in a range of different practice placements.

Available at https://www.nmc.org.uk/standards/standards-for-nurses/standards-of-proficiency-for-registered-nurses/nursing/practice-environment-case-studies-for-nursing-programmes/.

Chapter 7

Assessment and Feedback

Chapter Outline

INTRODUCTION

Assessment and feedback are the two elements that practice supervisors and practice assessors find most difficult or challenging when supporting students in practice. The two processes are closely linked. In order to provide feedback to a student you have to have made an assessment of what they did well and what they may have done less well. The purpose of this chapter is to explore the role of feedback in relation to the assessment process and the student learning experience. The strategies for assessing a student will be explored identifying

A Nurse's Survival Guide to Supervising and Assessing. https://doi.org/10.1016/B978-0-7020-8147-7.00007-7

how you can ensure that the assessment is evidence based, fair and objective. Feedback can be verbal or written, and can be formal or informal. Methods for giving feedback will be discussed by using the 'feedback sandwich' and how Pendleton's rules can be used.

It is the role of the practice supervisor to provide feedback to the student on their progress and whether they are demonstrating the skills, knowledge and attributes (professional behaviours) required to achieve their proficiencies. This helps both the practice supervisor and the student to identify what type of support and further learning opportunities the student may require to achieve specific proficiencies. It is the role of the practice assessor to collate the feedback provided by practice supervisors, service users and other people who have been involved in working with or supporting the student in order to make an assessment decision. This will include feedback on the student's performance and areas for improvement where required. The midpoint interview will be discussed as an example of when formal feedback is required. The chapter ends by looking at the importance of accurate documentation.

ASSESSMENT AND FEEDBACK

The assessment of pre-registration students can best be described as a 'process', with regular feedback to students being an integral aspect of this process. You should not have one without the other. High quality assessment will inform the feedback that students require enabling students to enhance their performance which will then be further assessed. Assessment in practice requires the collection of evidence upon which an assessment decision will be made.

WHAT IS ASSESSMENT?

Assessment in the context of nursing students in practice relates to the measure of a student's knowledge, skills and attributes (professional behaviours). It also includes the opportunity for the student to reflect on their own practice. The practice assessment document (PAD) structures the assessment process in practice and reflects three key stages of the assessment process.

> *Diagnostic assessment* – this relates to the initial interview which provides an opportunity to identify any learning needs the student may have. This may be based on feedback from previous placements or there could be areas that a student has identified, based on previous feedback or self-reflection. Reviewing the PAD and ongoing achievement record (OAR) is essential in identifying areas previously identified as a concern or requiring improvement. It is important to not only look at feedback from the last placement but all previous placements to identify any recurring patterns of concerns or areas for improvement. For students on their first placement it can be helpful to ask them for feedback from their participation in skills and simulation at university. It is

also a good opportunity to check out any prior healthcare experience they may have and any skills they have previously developed.

Formative assessment – this relates to the midpoint interview which provides the opportunity for the practice supervisor and assessor to provide feedback to the student on their progress and to identify any areas for further development. However, as feedback should be continuous the student should have received regular feedback prior to the formal formative assessment. Where causes for concern are present the academic assessor may also be involved at this stage and action plans developed.

Summative assessment – this relates to the final interview where the practice assessor will make a judgement on the student's progress and either confirm achievement and that the student has passed their placement or may make a decision that the student has not met the criteria for a pass in all the elements they have been assessed on and has failed the placement.

WHAT IS BEING ASSESSED?

The guide to what is being assessed is again the student's PAD. This contains the proficiencies, professional values/behaviours, and holistic assessments the student must be assessed upon during their placement.

It is the NMC that sets the standards of proficiency a student must have achieved for entry to the professional register. It is the practice supervisors/ assessors who are responsible for assessing these in practice. Their role is to judge the professional values and proficiencies of students using the assessment criteria detailed within the PAD. The different elements that must be assessed are:

● professional values/professional attitudes and behaviours
● proficiencies
● holistic assessments – episodes of care/in-placement assessments/medicines management.

While the document itself will have been produced by the university, the proficiency statements that need to be assessed will have been based upon the proficiencies set by the NMC. The proficiencies may be worded exactly the same as in the NMC *Standards of proficiency* (2018d) or may have been rephrased into new statements that include or two or more proficiencies. Holistic assessments will encompass a number of proficiencies and professional values all of which the student is required to achieve.

The practice supervisor is required to facilitate learning experiences related to the proficiencies and holistic assessments. They may, if agreed by the university and practice partner, also contribute to the student's assessment for some elements within the PAD. The practice assessor makes the overall assessment of the student's performance and that all elements have been met.

The focus for both supervisor and assessor is on the conduct, proficiency and achievement of the student they are supervising and/or assessing. Proficiencies encompass:

- knowledge
- skills
- attributes.

So, when assessing a student's progress the question to be asked is 'is the student demonstrating the expected level of knowledge and skills and the required attributes or professional behaviours expected of a nurse related to each element being assessed on their placement?'. For each element they must also consider whether the performance expectations they have of the student are appropriate for the stage/part of the programme they are on. Successful completion of a task within practice may not mean that a student is proficient.

Professional Values

The professional values/professional attitudes and behaviours may be identified separately in the PAD and will have been informed by the four sections of the NMC *Code* and also by the proficiencies in platform one - "Being an accountable professional" from the NMC *Standards of proficiency* (2018d) along with additional expectations of behaviours identified as important by the university and their practice partners. They are commonly presented as a list of statements that describe the behaviours the student must demonstrate in practice but may also be integrated into the proficiencies and holistic assessments. These can be useful for identifying behaviours related to a student's conduct such as punctuality or adherence to the dress code that can often be identified as a concern but do not relate directly to the NMC proficiencies. However, whilst some professional values will be innate, their application to nursing will take time to develop as they learn about the role of the nurse and develop a professional identity. An example of a professional value at two different stages/parts of a programme is:

> Part 1: The student maintains confidentiality in accordance with the NMC code.
> Part 3: The student maintains confidentiality in accordance with the NMC code and recognises limits to confidentiality, for example public interest and protection from harm (Pan London Practice Learning Group, 2019a).

The Proficiencies

The proficiencies in the PAD are statements that indicate what knowledge and skills the student is required to demonstrate. For example, a student may gather all the required information for an assessment but do they understand why the information is required and did they gain consent to undertake the assessment from the patient/service user? Also did they use the appropriate communication and relationship management skills when engaging with the patient/service user at a level of proficiency expected for the stage of their programme? An example of how a student's proficiency is expected to develop as they progress through their programme is shown below and are examples taken from the *All Wales Practice Assessment Document* and *Ongoing Achievement Record* (2020):

> Part 1: Begin to communicate effectively with colleagues and people with a range of mental, physical, cognitive and behavioural health challenges.
> Part 2: Use a range of skills and strategies to communicate with colleagues and people with a range of mental, physical, cognitive and behavioural health challenges.

Hopefully it is very clear that there is a much higher expectation of the range of communication skills a student would be expected to use in part 2 of their programme than in part 1.

Holistic Assessments

Holistic assessments require the student to demonstrate integration of knowledge, skills and professional behaviours to a given situation (care of a patient, care of a group of patients, medicines management or supporting and teaching a junior student/colleague). These require forward planning to identify an appropriate patient/service user group or learner and have identified proficiencies the student is required to achieve. It is essential to look at the learning outcomes to be achieved for each assessment as the level of proficiency and complexity of the patient/service user group increase in each part. For medicines management there is an increasing depth of knowledge expected of the student as they progress through each part of the programme.

> ! Ensure you are familiar with the PADs/OARs for the students that are on placement with you and discuss these with your colleagues so that everyone is clear regarding the standards expected of students.

SOURCES OF EVIDENCE TO INFORM THE ASSESSMENT DECISION

Unlike assessment of theory at the university which tends to focus primarily on written assessments, practice offers a wide range of assessment methods that are used collectively to make an overall assessment decision. The NMC (2018f) suggest that the following sources of evidence can be used to inform an assessment decision:

- direct observation of the student
- communication with practice supervisors

- student documentation, such as a PAD or ongoing record of achievement
- communication with any other practice assessors
- communication with anyone else who may be involved in the education of the student
- communication with the academic assessor
- student self-reflection
- communication, and an ongoing relationship, with the student.

In addition, practice assessors may also use:

- questioning skills to elicit a student's understanding of the theory underpinning a proficiency or skill
- production of materials or resources or a presentation that a student has developed in relation to one or more proficiencies
- feedback from service users
- the use of scenarios or a simulation in order to assess achievement of proficiencies that have not been available to a student or were not observed.

Criteria for a 'Good' Assessment

The NMC (2018f) have identified the three criteria that a sound assessment must meet. The assessments of a student must be:

- *Evidence based* – This means that it should use a range of evidence, for example direct observation, discussion, student reflections, completed documentation in the PAD and OAR, feedback from practice supervisors, service users and other people involved in the student's learning.
- *Objective* – This means that the assessment takes into consideration different learning styles, cultural backgrounds and communication styles and any reasonable adjustments the student may require.
- *Fair* – The assessment process must be transparent; it should be clearly documented within the PAD/OAR and utilise a variety of viewpoints. The student should be informed of the assessment decision in a timely manner and the reasons for the decision should be clear. The outcome, if it is the final assessment decision at the end of a placement, should never be a surprise to the student.

WHO IS THE ASSESSOR?

Each university will have made a decision with their practice partners regarding the roles of the practice supervisor and the practice assessor in the assessment process. This includes which elements within the PAD must be signed off by the practice assessor and which can be signed off by the practice supervisor. This is in line with the NMC Standards of student supervision and assessment (SSSA) Standards (2018b) which allows the practice supervisor to contribute to student assessment and identifies the role of the practice assessor as being responsible for assessing the overall performance of the student and ensuring that all relevant elements have been met. This includes:

- conducting assessments to confirm student achievement of proficiencies and programme outcomes for practice learning
- using feedback from practice supervisors to inform the assessment decision
- drawing on student records, direct observations, student self-reflection and other resources to make an assessment (NMC, 2018d).

The practice assessor does not need to be based in the same placement as the student, but they will need to have sufficient opportunities to observe the student in practice in order to make an overall assessment decision. This should occur across the length of the placement (or placements) not just at the end of the placement. If the practice assessor is not required to sign off all elements within the PAD, they will need to collate the information related to the student's performance using the range of evidence listed earlier. Where a practice assessor is supporting a student at a progression point, they will also work in partnership with the academic assessor to make recommendations for progression.

The role that feedback from practice supervisors and other relevant people plays in informing the practice assessor's decision highlights the importance of feedback in the assessment process.

WHAT IS FEEDBACK?

Feedback is often viewed as the giving of views, opinions or judgements about one to another. It should be based on past events and used to inform future behaviours. However, this implies a one-way process. Whilst it may provide students with information regarding their performance in practice, it may fail to engage the student fully in the process, so that they become a passive recipient in the process. This one-way transmission may reflect a perceived power imbalance between the student and the practice assessor which is strengthened by the assessor's power to pass or fail the student. If feedback is to have value and encourage development in the student's performance, the feedback process should always be constructive and based on evidence. This can then be used to inform a collaborative discussion exploring areas of strength and areas for further development. The student is provided with the opportunity to share their own views, ideas and solutions.

The aim of feedback is to provide the student with guidance on their performance and should therefore be directly related to the student's learning. If feedback is given too late or fails to focus on student performance, it will not be of benefit to the student. In fact, any feedback that fails to focus on a student's performance and development or that is not linked to the professional values and proficiencies they are required to achieve is unlikely to be valued.

FEEDBACK FOR STUDENTS

For many nurses, giving feedback to students can be challenging and probably the most difficult aspect of their role as a practice supervisor or assessor particularly where a student is underperforming. It is not uncommon for even experienced practice supervisors or assessors to be nervous about giving a student feedback regarding their performance, particularly when the feedback may not be viewed by the student as positive (Duffy, 2013). Unfortunately, sometimes opportunities for feedback are avoided due to fears of receiving a negative response or over-reaction by the student or if feedback is provided it lacks the detail the student needs to make improvements. Added to this, the pressures that exist in the clinical environment can impact on the timing and quality of feedback given. If the feedback is rushed, this can then cause problems later on if the student is unaware of the need for improvement or an action plan has not been agreed.

If feedback has not been consistent throughout the placement, students may be confused regarding the decisions that are made at the end of the placement especially if the evidence supporting those decisions is unclear. The NMC *Code* (2018a) requires all registrants to '*provide honest, accurate and constructive feedback to colleagues*' (9.1) and the responsibility of practice supervisors and practice assessors to provide feedback is clearly stated in the NMC Standards for all nursing, nursing associate and midwifery programmes. Research on feedback in nursing programmes has identified that students want and need feedback. However, students have reported that it is not always given or is not provided in a way that they recognise or understand in order for it to help them improve their performance (Calleja et al., 2016; Adamson et al., 2018; Ossenberg et al., 2019).

It is important to remember that feedback is not only about its value to the student, but it is also about ensuring the safety of patients and service users who are the recipients of care given by students. Where a student is not provided with feedback regarding poor performance there are potential risks to the people they care for.

Feedback requires a number of factors to be in place to be effective. It takes both confidence and skill to deliver feedback in a way that is helpful to the student. Feedback also needs to take place at the right time and in the right environment. When providing feedback it is important to provide time to allow for reflection on performance, sharing feedback and documenting a student's progress and any areas for improvement or actions required as they are all essential steps in the assessment process which must be followed if the student is to be given every opportunity to improve.

If any of these elements are lacking, then it is likely that the feedback experience will be unsatisfactory for everyone involved. Failure to provide feedback to students is a failure to follow the NMC *Code* (2018a) and the professional responsibilities set out in the NMC SSSA Standards (NMC, 2018b) and is an essential part of the assessment process as identified above. If there is no evidence of feedback provided to a student identifying areas for improvement and a decision is then made to fail the student, this would be judged as 'unfair' and due process would not have been followed. We will explore this further in Chapter 8.

Constructive Feedback

As highlighted above it is an NMC requirement that feedback is constructive and this applies regardless as to whether it is formal or informal. Lack of clarity in feedback can have a detrimental effect on the relationship between a student and their practice supervisor or assessor and can compromise the self-esteem for all involved. Constructive feedback is:

- objective
- non-judgemental
- based on specific evidence
- motivating
- encourages discussion
- allows for a positive course to be set for the future
- boosts student confidence
- encourages future learning.

There are many benefits to providing constructive feedback to students as it provides opportunities to share examples of good practice, enhances their learning and allows students the opportunity to reflect on their practice. Spontaneous feedback is especially valuable as it provides a platform for a student to undertake self-reflection of their performance in the moment and can provide valuable insight into the student's perception of their own ability. For this reason self-reflection should be encouraged in feedback situations. The student's self-reflection should also provide opportunities for a clear discussion on strengths and weaknesses, and help students to plan further learning experiences. Without clarity of feedback, students risk engaging in reflective exercises that are not related to the development of clinical competence and as a result may miss potential learning experiences.

Students Want Feedback

Students value constructive feedback and define this as an attribute of a 'good' practice supervisor or practice assessor. Where a student receives little or no feedback or it is not delivered in a supportive way then the student is likely to evaluate their experience in practice poorly. Feedback is important to students because they want to know your opinion regarding their performance on clinical placement. No student wants to fail their placement and for this reason they can become preoccupied with receiving feedback about their performance. It is easy to understand why feedback is so important to a student as not only can it provide reassurance on current achievements; it also provides an opportunity to improve if there are any deficits or problems identified. Students rely on the practice supervisor and practice assessor to tell them of any concerns regarding their performance so that they can make improvements if required. If a student hears nothing, then unless indicated otherwise, they will conclude that they are doing well and should have no cause for concern.

While feedback is a vital component of a fair and objective assessment, it is important to ensure that students, who can feel quite vulnerable, are protected and their self-esteem is not damaged as a consequence of the feedback given. As a result, feedback can become a delicate balancing act between protecting a student's feelings and being honest, which can be quite daunting. In order to address these issues, it is important to have a clear understanding of the feedback to be provided, the evidence to support any areas for concern and a plan for how the feedback can be delivered in a supportive and developmental way.

WHEN SHOULD FEEDBACK BE PROVIDED?

Feedback should be a continuous process. Whilst there are key points identified in the student's PAD students should ideally receive feedback each time that they are in practice and certainly whenever any individual professional values, skills or proficiencies are signed off. Feedback that is unplanned is called informal feedback.

Informal Feedback

Informal feedback can occur any time throughout a clinical placement and is usually given in response to a specific event. It can happen at any time and is generally unplanned. This is more likely to occur between a practice supervisor and student as time with the practice assessor is likely to be more focussed on assessing specific proficiencies or undertaking an episode of care or in-placement assessment. Informal feedback may take place on-the-spot or as an informal conversation after an event or situation occurs in practice. In general, the earlier in a placement that informal feedback becomes routine between the practice supervisor and student the better. Establishing frequent and spontaneous lines of communication will be of benefit to both the practice supervisor and student and help in developing a positive relation between the two. Insufficient feedback can have a negative impact on the student learning experience, resulting in increased anxiety and insecurity during clinical placement as they have no idea if they are performing well or not. However, if feedback is regularly given then it can be used to support the student's learning and provide valuable opportunities for reflection.

Practice supervisors also benefit from providing students with regular feedback, as it helps in developing confidence in discussing a student's progress with them. Keep in mind that either the practice supervisor or the student can instigate feedback; it is not simply the responsibility of the practice supervisor.

Some students may repeatedly request feedback. If this becomes excessive then it may indicate under confidence so understanding why they are constantly seeking feedback is important and agreeing when it is appropriate, for example after they have engaged in a new activity or when undertaking an activity they had been trying to improve upon following previous feedback. Agreeing specific time periods where this may be possible can allay their concerns. It's also a good idea to put a time limit on the discussions to ensure the time used is focused.

Try to seize these opportunities when students request feedback to provide them with an honest and useful answer. If they broach the subject then they want to hear your answer and this is a great time to give accurate feedback and also to further probe the student's understanding of what has been happening. However, where a student is reluctant to receive feedback it is important to ensure that the feedback relates to the student's learning outcomes and is non-threatening. It does not need to be lengthy; a quick summary highlighting what the student did well and areas that the student needs to work on which will be discussed at a future planned meeting lets them know that their practice is being observed and that the practice supervisor/assessor are engaging with the assessment process.

Formative feedback can help students to rate their clinical performance more realistically. If students are not reaching the required standard then feedback should be more frequent to provide the student with opportunities to develop and improve. However, take care to ensure that you are not overdoing your feedback, as students may feel overwhelmed.

Unfortunately it is not unusual for informal feedback to only be used when there is a concern regarding a student's performance. Students who are doing well and achieving all their proficiencies outcomes may miss out on feedback because they are seen to be 'doing OK'. It is quite common to find that feedback is associated with poor performance, rather than being used as a tool to encourage achievement. Typically, it is the informal feedback that students will be denied if they are producing a satisfactory performance. However, there is great value in delivering simple and frequent praise for students who are achieving. Not only is this a great boost to self-esteem but it will also make the overall assessment more credible if it is made obvious that the student's performance is being reviewed as a whole rather than picking on isolated events.

If a student is doing well on their placement but does not receive any feedback then they will worry. Equally if informal feedback is not used to identify areas where a student needs to improve their performance then they may believe that all is well and will be devastated at the formal feedback events if they are then told they are not meeting the required standard.

> ! Informal feedback is as important as formal feedback. It is flexible and can range from immediate on-the-spot feedback, or be delivered as a summary of the student's performance at the end of the day. Feedback should take place as close to an event as possible to ensure relevance and accuracy of reflection.

Formal Feedback

Formal feedback is the feedback that must take place as part of the assessment process and the occasions these must take place will be identified in the PAD. In general formal feedback must be provided at the midpoint and final interviews. It is also required after the completion of any of the holistic assessments such as the episodes of care, in-point assessments or the assessments related to medicines management. It is the role of the practice assessor to provide formal feedback on these occasions. Formal feedback should therefore be a planned event. It should be structured and ideally be conducted in a quiet area away from the noise and distraction of the practice environment. It is very important that privacy is ensured and that adequate time is allowed for the feedback to be detailed enough that the student can understand it. Formal feedback can be more challenging than informal feedback if the feedback highlights any concerns regarding underperformance by the student. This will need to be documented in the student's PAD and this feedback will be used to inform the final decision as to whether the student has passed or failed their placement.

For this reason formal feedback events should never be 'sprung' on a student without prior warning. The focus of the meeting should always be planned in order to make the best use of the time. If these events are not planned then the feedback may be unclear or not be based on feedback from other staff involved in supporting the student. This will only increase student insecurity and anxiety. The student also needs time to prepare themselves for the feedback event. Students who are not given sufficient warning of a formal interview may feel quite intimidated, and reluctant to voice their opinions or concerns. A lack of two-way interaction will jeopardise the interaction needed for insight and development. Keep in mind that if a student enters a formal interview feeling negative for any reason then the time you spend with them will be of little benefit.

When planning for formal feedback the following points need to be considered:

- Set the time and date with the student for all formal feedback.
- Ensure the student has plenty of opportunity to prepare for it.
- Where possible identify with the student what the focus of the interview will be on.
- Ask the student to consider what they want to discuss at the meeting.

Regardless of what type of feedback is being given it is important to remember that it must be clear and unambiguous. Too little information and the student may be unsure of what is being said and what is required of them or how this relates to their proficiencies. When information is withheld, then feedback becomes a superficial exercise and will be of little value to a student. If feedback includes too much information the student may feel overwhelmed, taking in little of what has actually been said. Feedback should always include examples from practice and should also include specific targets and standards. If the feedback is not clear then ultimately the student may lack direction. By linking the feedback to evidence, with specific examples of events that have taken place in practice, the student will have a clearer understanding of what they need to do to improve their performance.

It is likely that the first opportunity for formal feedback is the midpoint assessment. We will look at that in more detail next as a poorly managed midpoint assessment will lead to significant problems later on if there are concerns regarding the student's performance.

THE MIDPOINT INTERVIEW

The main purpose of the midpoint interview is to discuss with the student their progress and performance to date. This will include proficiencies achieved, identifying strengths and areas for development, and identifying what other proficiencies still need to be achieved including any of the episodes of care or in-placement assessments. The midpoint interview is a key step in the assessment process, allowing both the practice assessor and the student the chance to look back on what they have achieved during the preceding weeks, and to plan for what still needs to be done. At this stage, both the practice assessor and the student should have an insight into whether or not the required level of performance is likely to be achieved within the time remaining.

During the first part of the placement the practice assessor must have had opportunities to have worked with the student in order to make an assessment of the student's performance. Depending on the decision by the university the practice supervisor may have signed off individual proficiencies and the professional values for the midpoint. At some point however, it is important to take stock of how far the student has come on their learning journey. Time out will need to be taken to review the progress made, reflect on the positives and areas that require improvement and plan for the 'second half'. Areas for improvement may also include better support and feedback to the student; it is not just a focus on how well the student has done, or not. The midpoint interview represents half time. It is a time to evaluate, regroup and refocus. It is a time to review the initial learning plan and decide whether this has been effective. It is the time to ask questions such as:

- Have the goals set at the initial interview been achieved?
- Have the different aspects of the learning plan worked in the way they were designed to?
- Were any changes made to the plan and why?
- What still needs to be done in order to achieve the desired goals?
- What needs to be done to enable the student to get to where they need to be by the end of the placement?

The midpoint interview is a time to re-energise, re-motivate and spur the student on to achieve more in the second half of the practice placement.

Purpose of the Midpoint Interview

Although the midpoint interview is a formal step in the assessment process, it is a formative rather than a summative component of assessment. The purpose of the midpoint interview is to identify and provide information that can be used effectively to improve the student's learning rather than to test whether specific proficiencies have been achieved. The midpoint interview is measuring how far the student has progressed towards achieving the set goals, identifying their successes and where they may be having difficulties. This information can then be used to make necessary adjustments to their learning plan, such as the student spending more time with their practice supervisor or identifying and/or offering alternative or further opportunities for specific practice learning opportunities. The feedback given as part of the midpoint interview should help the student become aware of any gaps that exist between the desired goal and their current knowledge, understanding or skills and guide them through the actions necessary to achieve that goal. The purpose of formative feedback is to enhance learning, not to pass judgement. The key function of the midpoint interview therefore is to inform both the practice assessor and the student about what has already been learnt and what still needs to be achieved.

When Should the Midpoint Interview Take Place?

The midpoint interview needs to take place at a point in the student's placement that will allow plenty of time and opportunity for them to address any areas for development. There has to be time for the student to participate in the necessary learning experiences, practise and refine skills if they are to gain the level of proficiency required. The ideal therefore is to time the midpoint interview at a point in the placement where progress can be properly established and advice given in a timely manner.

This may sound obvious but it is not uncommon for the university to be contacted to be informed that a student is about to fail their placement and when the situation is discussed it is found that the midpoint assessment took place very late and the student has not been given sufficient time to make the improvements required which makes the assessment unfair and invalid.

The midpoint interview should therefore always take place as close as possible to the midpoint of the student's time on placement. Too early and insufficient information and evidence will have been gathered; too late and there is insufficient time for the student to be given the opportunity to improve. If it is a short placement this can be more problematic and there is little lee-way in deciding the date.

The date for the midpoint interview should always be agreed at the initial interview as this ensures it takes place on time. Try to select a day when the placement may be less busy, if that is possible, and ensure the off-duty is planned for both the student and practice assessor to be on duty on the agreed date.

The length of time required to undertake the interview will depend on how well the student is progressing. If there are concerns regarding the student's performance more time may be required and the Link Lecturer or academic assessor may also need to be invited. Regardless of whether the student is progressing well or not a suitable space to hold the interview must be found that is free from interruptions.

Preparing for the Midpoint Interview

The practice assessor will need to gather the evidence upon which the feedback will be based. The different sources of evidence were listed earlier in this chapter. In addition the practice assessor will need to plan time to seek feedback from the practice supervisor(s) and any other staff involved in supporting the students. Ideally their feedback should be documented in the PAD but clarification with them may be needed if the evidence they have documented is unclear or to check if there are any updates to what has been recorded. This means that the practice assessor needs time to review all the evidence in the PAD BEFORE the meeting occurs. If the student has an e-PAD this will be easier as it is accessible anytime. If it is a paper PAD the practice assessor will need to be given it in advance of the meeting to provide time to review what has been recorded which requires advance preparation. Let's look at what happens when a practice assessor fails to prepare for the midpoint interview and then at an organised and well-prepared practice assessor.

A Poor Midpoint Interview

Carol the practice assessor failed to plan for the midpoint interview and 6 weeks into the 8-week placement the student, Gina, reminds her. Carol quickly arranges a date and time to meet and Gina brings her PAD to the meeting.

> Carol (reading the PAD): *'So it's about student progress. Right! So, how are you progressing?'*
> Gina: *'I'm really enjoying it. I'm having a great time. Everybody is really friendly and, you know, I can do stuff. I'm meeting people and …'*
> Carol (butting in): *'Good and you feel you are learning and everything?'*
> Gina: *'Yeh! Yeh'*
> Carol: *'Thats good! I know I haven't had many opportunities to observe you in practice, well only a couple of times really, but I've not heard anything bad about you so that's good isn't it! I can see some of your proficiencies have been signed off so that is good isn't it. All being well you should get through the placement without any problems. So everything's fine then!'*

A Good Midpoint Interview

In this scenario Daniel, the practice assessor, arranged the date for the midpoint interview at the initial interview with the student, Kelly. He has reviewed the

PAD before the meeting and managed to talk with the practice supervisor who has been supporting Kelly.

> Daniel: *'It's great to have this time to review the placement with you because we had the initial interview in the first week, didn't we? And we went through the different proficiencies you wanted to achieve. So just to recap, we identified 13 proficiencies that you could achieve here and there are two extra that you particularly wanted to achieve. So we will go through these in the next half hour. Just so you know I have talked to Gill your practice supervisor and some of the other staff you have been working with to get their feedback. Although I have had a few opportunities to work with you I've talked to some of the other staff to get their feedback on how you've been doing and it's been really useful to get other people's viewpoints. So I'll let you know what they said in a moment. Is that OK?'*
> Kelly: *'Yes. Thank you'.*
> Daniel: *'So, before I do that tell me how you feel you are progressing and what has gone well'*

There are clearly very big differences in the way Carol and Daniel conduct the interview. Daniel sets out a clear agenda for the meeting and knows exactly what needs to be done. He appears to have prepared for the interview. Carol on the other hand doesn't seem very sure about what is involved. Daniel demonstrates he knows exactly what the purpose of the meeting is – to review Kelly's progress. He starts by revisiting the initial interview and learning plan. The initial interview is a good starting point for discussing progress. It is useful to remind students about the goals that were agreed and about how they felt and what they seemed anxious about. In the time between initial and midpoint interviews students can forget where they started and can focus too much on problems or worries that have arisen during the placement. As they gain competence and confidence they can forget what they didn't know and/or couldn't do so are unaware of the progress they have made. It is therefore important to point out exactly where progress has been made and remind the student about what they thought they didn't know or couldn't do at the start of the placement and the situations where they lacked confidence.

In both scenarios, the practice assessors start by asking the student to comment on their own progress. It is important to allow the student to assess their own learning, as self-assessment helps the student to take ownership of their learning and take some control over the way they meet their learning needs. It is important to remind your student of the ultimate goal of the placement and encourage them to articulate the progress they feel they have made so far. Skilful questioning can help learners identify any barriers to learning they are experiencing as well as enabling them to clarify any areas of misunderstanding that may have arisen. Daniel's approach is to refocus on the goals set in the initial interview, encouraging Kelly to reflect on how she is progressing towards achieving each one. By asking Kelly to describe her progress he is enabling her to reflect and acknowledge her achievements.

Celebrating Success

It is vital that success and achievement are recognised at the midpoint interview as this helps motivate the student to strive for higher goals. Helping the student get a sense of their progress requires prompts to help them to recall what they could do or knew at the start of the placement. Reflecting back to where they started and comparing this with where they are now helps students to appreciate the range and complexity of learning to date. This is especially important for students who have made good progress in some areas but not in others. It is important to remember as highlighted in Chapter 6 that each student will have a different style and capacity to learn. Some students will be practical hands-on learners who will acquire psychomotor skills easily. Others will be able to discuss the rationale for care and excel in decision-making activities, whilst others will be good communicators, demonstrating the empathy and caring aspects of nursing naturally and easily. It is therefore important when celebrating the student's achievements to remind them that 'practice-based' learning requires the integration of knowledge and skills with praxis. that is, putting theory into action.

Measuring Progress at the Midpoint

It is important to compare the student's achievement at the midpoint interview with what they were expected to achieve. If goals or targets have not been met, explore the reasons for this. Consider whether the goals set were realistic given the time and opportunities available to the student. It is also important to discuss any specific problems the student may have encountered, for example accessing the necessary patient care experiences.

It is also crucial to clearly articulate to the student any areas that need addressing. As discussed earlier, what you think you have said is not always what the student hears. Use clear language avoiding euphemisms and check the student has understood. However, try to use non-evaluative language if possible, for example 'Have you thought about asking the patient…?' rather than 'Your questioning of the patient was inadequate'. When highlighting weaknesses it is important to avoid generalisations. Give the student specific examples: '*remember last Tuesday when we were completing the admission interview with Mr Sing I had to remind you to ask him about … and again on Friday with Mr Short*' rather than '*there have been lots of times when we have been working together when I have had to remind you to ask ….*' This will help the student view the comments in context and make it clearer what they need to improve on. Using examples to emphasise key points also helps to keep the interview constructive, objective and evidence based.

Using a feedback model could have enhanced the feedback by Carol particularly at the midpoint interview.

FEEDBACK MODELS

There are a number of feedback models which can be found in the literature and also available on the internet so exploring these models is useful as they often provide good examples of how they can be used. They all tend to have some core similarities, so you may wish to explore these to find one that works best for you. The one that is most commonly discussed is the feedback sandwich.

The Feedback Sandwich

The feedback sandwich is a very simple model to remember and an easy way of delivering both formal and informal feedback. It should consist of one specific area for improvement 'sandwiched' between two specific positives (or praises). It is a particularly useful technique when giving feedback to students with low self-esteem, as, when used correctly, it begins and ends with positive statements. In fact, a well-timed, well-targeted and well-constructed feedback sandwich will:

● encourage student learning
● motivate future learning
● reduce confusion
● improve self-esteem
● value the student's contribution to their learning.

Example of a Feedback Sandwich

Ehren is undertaking a placement in a care of the elderly ward. In his first week his practice supervisor has noticed that he is very keen to involve himself in all aspects of patient care but seems to avoid situations where he is required to deliver care to one particular patient who is confused and has frequent outbursts of verbal aggression. His practice supervisor decides to use a feedback sandwich to open up a discussion on Ehren's feelings related to this patient.

Praise

'Hi Ehren, I just wanted to say well done on your first week here, I'm really pleased with how well you are doing in getting involved in the care activities with the people you have been allocated to. I have noticed that you are very good at gaining their consent before you do anything and explaining what you are doing. I was very impressed when you approached Mrs Shah and recognised that she is partially deaf and so you ensured that you were facing her and took time to talk louder and more slowly to explain what you were going to do and checked she understood and consented. You're making really good progress towards achieving your proficiencies related to communication so well done'.

Concern

'I'm sorry about Mr Jones' verbal aggression. I could see by your reaction on Tuesday when he was yelling that you felt uncomfortable talking with him. Communicating effectively with people who are distressed or angry is an important skill to develop'.

Praise

'I'd like to work with you on that, as I have seen how much potential you have in communicating with the patients here. How would you feel about us developing a plan to communicate with Mr Jones and different approaches you might take so that you can develop your skills in that area?'

> ! The feedback sandwich is the easy way to remember how to deliver feedback constructively. It can identify improvements while maintaining a student's self-esteem.

Pendleton's Rules

This model developed by Pendleton et al. (1984), is popular in medical education. Its strength is that it is learner-centred and encourages critical reflection. It has a number of steps that can be used in nursing as follows:

- The student discusses what went well.
- The practice supervisor/assessor confirms what was done well and adds anything else the student did well.
- The student reflects on areas that did not go well and how they could be improved upon.
- The practice supervisor/assessor confirms those areas that did not go well and adds anything else that could be improved upon.
- An action plan is developed together and agreed upon. Ideally the student should identify the help they need but junior students or less confident senior students may need assistance in identifying the actions required.

This model can work well after a specific activity or event, although not if the activity did not go well as focussing on the positives when both parties know it did not go well will be difficult and may seem patronising. However, if there are positives to be found, helping the student to see that is important but in this situation the feedback sandwich may be a better option.

ARE YOU PREPARED FOR ASSESSMENT AND FEEDBACK?

The preparation of practice supervisors and assessors for undertaking assessments and delivering effective feedback to students is essential and should be part of the preparation for the role. However, it is not uncommon to find practice supervisors and assessors who lack confidence regarding assessment and feedback and need support to develop the skills in order to give fair and objective feedback. Universities along with employers run regular workshops to prepare staff for these roles or to update staff who need a refresher. These can be half or whole day events and may also be available on-line enabling staff to access them at a time that fits best for them.

Observing an experienced colleague providing feedback can be extremely valuable. However, this should only be undertaken with consent from the student and where it would be appropriate. Remember that students can feel vulnerable so more staff present can make them feel even more vulnerable but they may feel unable to say no. The student may feel more comfortable with this if the person attending is also their practice supervisor who knows them and can contribute to the discussion.

CHALLENGES GIVING FEEDBACK

There are a multitude of reasons as to why practice supervisors or assessors fail to deliver feedback. One of the most common issues are the time constraints and competing clinical pressures that can impact on the time that they can spend with students. Of course, the irony is that the really busy shifts tend to be the times that students require maximum support and feedback. In addition, sick leave, shift changes and annual leave can all impact on the availability of feedback opportunities for students; although with the roles of both practice supervisors and practice assessors available to support and feedback to students this should be less of a problem.

It is likely that most students will have very little appreciation that giving feedback may be difficult for some practice supervisors or assessor. As a result, they may assume that if you have any concerns about their progress then you will let them know and so no news is good news! While students are encouraged during their programme to reflect upon their own performance, it is unrealistic to expect that all students will be able to identify and rectify their own practice without the support and feedback of their practice supervisor and practice assessor.

> ! Ensure the student knows when you are giving them some feedback and ensure it is clear, constructive and timely.

Feedback About Concerns

There may be times where the feedback to be provided relates to concerns about the student's performance. The common areas where feedback may be more difficult include:

- feedback that confirms a student has failed an element or elements in the PAD
- students with very poor self-esteem who are not making satisfactory progress
- students who are unable to accept limitations in their competence.

In such situations it is important to seek help in delivering the feedback. For example, in some situations the practice supervisor may be considered, especially if the student has built a rapport with this person. However, there is the risk with this approach that a student may consider that 'everyone' in the practice area is ganging up on them.

Link Lecturers may also be consulted for difficult feedback situations, and sometimes a student may appreciate having a university lecturer present for support. At other times students may perceive this action as 'bringing in the big guns' and be even more intimidated by this outcome.

If the feedback is being provided for the purpose of improving student performance it is important that the student understands what the concern is as they cannot improve their performance if they do not understand what the issue is. As discussed throughout this chapter feedback must be specific and linked to evidence. For this reason it is vital that once feedback has been delivered that the student's understanding of what has been discussed is checked in case they have misunderstood the concerns being raised and so enable any misconceptions to be corrected. It is important to remember that the feedback given may not always be the same as the feedback received, so encourage students to reflect on the feedback provided and outline their interpretation of its content.

> ! Always check that the student understands the feedback they have been given, how this relates to their proficiencies and professional values and what actions are needed to improve performance.

Where there are significant concerns about a student's performance that are likely to result in the student failing practice the student's academic assessor must be informed and the concerns discussed. If it is agreed that the student is not meeting the required standard then either the academic assessor or Link Lecturer will attend the final feedback meeting to provide support to both the student and the practice assessor and ensure a fair assessment takes place. Chapter 8 will discuss supporting the underperforming student in more detail.

The key to delivering difficult feedback is to access the most appropriate support and then deliver the feedback as professionally as possible. Avoiding difficult feedback is not, and will never be, the solution.

FEEDBACK AND STUDENT SELF-ESTEEM

While you may deliver feedback in an honest and encouraging way this will not always ensure that a student responds positively to your feedback. Although it is reasonable to assume that honesty is important, a student may not interpret the feedback as encouraging if they are vulnerable due to low self-esteem. In fact, students with low self-esteem may have a fear of negative evaluation and avoid feedback situations as a way of coping. While students with high self-esteem may view feedback as an opportunity to improve, those with low self-esteem may see it as threatening and therefore the feedback needs to be carefully handled.

For this reason, you must always ensure that you deliver feedback which comments on positive aspects in order to maintain or improve self-esteem. This approach will be fairly simple when providing praise for students who are performing well and reaching a high standard; however, it can be difficult when feedback includes comment on poor performance. It is important therefore to be aware of non-verbal cues that might tell you that the student is finding the feedback meeting difficult or is having difficulties in understanding what you are saying. Check their understanding of the feedback that has been given and clarify anything they have not understood or are unclear about. Remember to use the evidence gathered as the basis for the discussion and clarify terminology used if the student is unclear. Always try to link the feedback to the professional values, proficiencies or additional holistic assessments so that the student understands what the feedback relates to. Feedback must always be related to the student's work performance and never based on the character of the student.

! The self-esteem of students must be taken into account when delivering feedback. Feedback should be directly related to specific proficiencies and professional values and not directed towards personal attributes or a student's character.

DOCUMENTING FEEDBACK

Documenting feedback that is concise but covers everything that needs to be recorded is essential as this information will need to be used for future meetings with the student. If documenting the midpoint interview for example, then this will be used as a basis for the final interview. Documented feedback must include both strengths and areas for improvement the student needs to develop further as they progress through their programme. Documentation of feedback is often an area that practice assessors struggle with especially if there are concerns about a student's performance. They may try to play down any concerns when writing about them as they are concerned with the fact that what they write is permanently recorded in the student's assessment document and also because students can become distressed about what is written. It is not unusual for students to discourage their practice assessors from documenting feedback that identifies areas of concern. It is an NMC requirement that decisions about a student's assessment are clearly documented in order that they can be used across the different placements a student will undertake and also are available to the academic assessor who will use the information provided to make the decision regarding a student's progression in conjunction with the practice assessor (NMC, 2018f). Documenting feedback to students also falls under the NMC *Code* (NMC, 2018a) which requires *clear and accurate records* to be kept which includes the student's PAD, not just patient records.

The NMC *Code* (2018a) states that you must:

10.1 complete all records at the time or as soon as possible after an event, recording if the notes are written some time after the event

10.2 identify any risks or problems that have arisen and the steps taken to deal with them, so that colleagues who use the records have all the information they need

10.3 complete all records accurately and without any falsification

10.4 attribute any entries you make in any paper or electronic records to yourself, making sure they are clearly written, dated and timed, and do not include unnecessary abbreviations, jargon or speculation.

The professional obligation here is clear. As a registered nurse the practice assessor is accountable and responsible for the assessment decision they make about a student nurse. It is important therefore to ensure that the PAD provides clear and accurate records of events during the student's practice placement. The clearer and more specific the documentation is, the more clarity there will be to support the steps that have been taken in the assessment process. Documented feedback will contribute to the 'audit trail' within the practice placement and provide evidence that supports the decision to pass or fail a student.

Occasionally a student may make a formal appeal against the outcome of a failed practice assessment. The documentation in the PAD/OAR will be used to determine whether an evidence-based, objective and fair assessment took place.

What Needs to Be Documented?

First, let's return to the examples of the midpoint interviews discussed earlier in this chapter and see what Carol and Daniel wrote in their student's PADs.

Carol: *'Gina has settled into the ward well and is making good progress with her learning outcomes. Although I have not had much opportunity to work with her my colleagues have found her to be a willing worker and learner'.*

Daniel: *'Kelly is improving slowly. She is motivated and eager to participate in care activities. She is aware now of emergency procedures and where we keep equipment on the ward. Her nursing care is safe and she has received positive feedback from service users. She has made progress towards achieving several of her outcomes and has achieved 10 so far. A key area to focus on now is her general knowledge of medications related to the service users she is caring for and she needs to understand the rationale behind the accurate charting of food and fluid charts for some of our service users. She is improving with her time management but still needs to organise her work so she finishes it all on time. We have agreed action plans to address these areas'.*

The comments provided by Daniel give a clear indication of the progress made by Kelly, celebrating her achievements. He also identifies clearly Kelly's areas for improvement. In contrast, Carol's comments do not tell us what Gina has or has not achieved. There is nothing in this account that can be used to measure Gina's progress over the remaining weeks. We do not know what outcomes have been achieved and which are outstanding. There is nothing in this account to provide guidance to Gina of how to progress further. Sadly this type of feedback is often seen.

The documentation of feedback must be evidence based, objective and fair. It must also reflect any verbal discussions that took place with the student. A summary of any discussions that took place must be recorded and must be factual. Documented feedback must not be kept from the student or written in secret, nor should it ever appear in notes or letters that do not form part of the assessment documentation. If this happens the student will interpret this as collaborating against them rather than working with them.

It is important to resist the temptation to dilute the written feedback in order to spare a student's feelings as this will result in an inaccurate recording of events. In fact, a discrepancy between what is said and what is written only increases student anxiety, as a non-specific report can seriously undermine student confidence. Written feedback should also be dated and signed by the practice assessor and the student as it often forms the basis of an action plan. It may be helpful to use the feedback sandwich for the written documentation as this will ensure that this reflects the approach used at the feedback meeting. If an action plan has been developed this must be clearly signposted. If the feedback is clearly written then the student can use the documentation to discuss their learning needs with their practice supervisor, their academic assessor and also with practice supervisors, assessors, and lecturers on future placements.

! All feedback must be recorded in the student's PAD. Remember that if it isn't written down, there will be no evidence that feedback has been provided.

DOCUMENTING THE ONGOING ACHIEVEMENT RECORD

It is an NMC requirement that there is an ongoing record of the student's achievement across the length of their programme. This record of a student's progress must be made available from one placement to the next (this may be combined PAD/OAR or the PAD and OAR as two separate documents). The practice assessor will need to complete all required sections in the PAD/OAR at the final interview. This record should provide a brief summary of the placement and clearly identify the student's strengths and any areas that require further development in subsequent placements.

The PAD/OAR should not contain any information that has not been discussed with the student during the placement; rather it should be a summary of events and the discussions that have taken place during the placement. This information will be invaluable to the student and subsequent practice supervisors and practice assessors to chart the student's progress and will help identify any areas that require particular development plans on future placements. Without this information the student's progress through their learning experiences could be compromised and it denies them the opportunity to improve their performance with support on future placements.

Action Points

- Reflect on your experience of providing feedback to students and keep this in your NMC Revalidation folder to discuss at your next Revalidation meeting.
- Try to set a 'feedback schedule' at the beginning of the placement to ensure you keep to the timeframes required and the student is aware when to expect it.
- Identify students who are vulnerable or display low self-esteem and moderate your feedback accordingly.
- Practice using the feedback sandwich every time you deliver feedback to students and staff – practice makes perfect!

Chapter 8

Supporting the Student Who Is Not Making the Progress Expected

Chapter Outline

INTRODUCTION

The purpose of this chapter is to explore the skills required in supporting a student who is not making the progress expected, and the actions that can be taken to support them to improve their performance. It will look at the warning signs that can alert the practice supervisor and practice assessor that the student is underperforming and may not be able to demonstrate achievement of their proficiencies. Accessing help when an underperforming student is identified is essential, and can ensure that both the staff in practice and the student are appropriately supported. Action plans are an important part of the assessment process and make explicit the expectations of the student to improve their performance and ensures the support available to them is made clear. They also provide evidence of the actions taken and are an important tool for communicating with all staff involved in supporting the student. Unfortunately, despite the evidence, some practice assessors will fail to fail the student. The reasons for this are explored, including the coercive strategies that may be used by some students.

THE CHALLENGES IN SUPPORTING A STUDENT WHO IS NOT MAKING THE PROGRESS EXPECTED

Supporting a student who is not making the progress expected can be very difficult for many staff in practice. The nature of the event means that it is never a pleasant experience, and can be equally difficult for supervisors, assessors, and students alike. Supporting students who are not achieving the expected level of proficiency or not demonstrating the required professional values requires everyone involved to ensure that due process is followed and that the final assessment decision is evidence-based, fair and objective.

The supporting information for the Standards of student supervision and assessment (SSSA), provided by the Nursing and Midwifery Council (NMC) (2018f) on their website, has a section that focuses on 'students who are not meeting the progress expected'. This is a change in terminology, with a move away from a previous focus on failure to fail. The word *fail* is a highly emotive word. No one likes to be told they are failing, and being told you may fail can be both frightening and threatening to a student. This change in terminology has the potential to alter the approach by practice supervisors and practice assessors when supporting a student who is not making the progress expected. Whilst the term *fail* is used when a student has not passed their practice, many universities use the term *referred* to describe a student who has not met the required standard for one or more proficiencies in their practice assessment at their first attempt. A student is only deemed to have failed when it is their final attempt at an assessment. Terminology is important, as it can change the way both practice assessors and students view the assessment process.

IDENTIFYING UNDERPERFORMANCE

When faced with a student who is not meeting the required standards for the proficiencies and professional values in their practice assessment document

(PAD), the first step is to ascertain exactly what it is that the student is not achieving and why. This must be done as soon as concerns are first identified.

A student can only be considered to be underperforming during a practice placement if they are falling short of the standard set by the NMC proficiencies and professional values that they are attempting on that placement. These are the only aspects of the student's performance that a practice supervisor/assessor is required to assess. This means that if it is believed that a student is not reaching the required standard of performance expected, then the concerns must be related to one or more specific proficiencies or professional values within their assessment document. Where a student's performance is causing concerns, but it is difficult to identify how this relates to the professional values or proficiencies, it is important to seek advice from the Link Lecturer or academic assessor as a matter of urgency.

If a thorough initial interview was undertaken at the beginning of the placement, then identifying a student who is not making the expected progress against the identified elements to be assessed should be relatively simple. Clear identification of the different assessment elements that the student would be expected to focus on and how they will demonstrate having achieved them should have been agreed at the initial interview. Clarity over what is expected will ensure that the practice supervisor, the practice assessor and the student will be able to identify when the student's practice falls short of this standard.

It is important to always check that what is expected of the student is appropriate for the stage of the programme they are on and reflects the requirements set out in the proficiency statement, professional value or any of the holistic assessments.

WHY IS THE STUDENT NOT MAKING THE PROGRESS EXPECTED?

Causes for underperformance by a student may be external to them or internal to them. Causes that are external to them identified by the Pan London Practice Learning Group (2019b, p. 3) are:

- *Unclear expectations* – this can relate to the lack of understanding by the practice supervisor or assessor about what the student is permitted to do or should be doing. This may arise due to a poor initial interview or a lack of understanding of the requirements in the PAD. It may also reflect unclear expectations by the student as to what they are required to do, especially on their first placement.
- *Insufficient support* – if the student feels unsupported this can impact on their motivation to learn; it can also mean that they are unable to get the support they require to make the required progress.
- *Working relationships or culture of setting* – very busy settings or settings that are very different to the type of placements experienced before can leave a student feeling lost or insecure: A&E, critical care units, prisons, secure

mental health services. Environments where students are not made welcome, and where they feel excluded by staff, will leave the student feeling isolated and unable to access support.

● *Poor communication amongst staff* – this can impact on students if a practice supervisor has not kept colleagues informed about the student's progress or learning needs or ensured that the student is supported when they are not on duty.

● *Insufficient feedback from supervisors or assessors* – without feedback students do not have a clear understanding of whether they are making the required progress, or what improvements they need to make. This can cause significant concerns for students.

● Causes for underperformance that are internal to the student may be:

● *Lack of interest in setting / working environment* – some placements may be unpopular with students due to the client group within the setting, or they are not seen as meeting their personal long-term career goal.

● *Stress and pressure* – in addition to learning in practice, students have academic assessments to complete as well as external pressures related to family responsibilities. If they have previously been unsuccessful on a placement there is an additional pressure on them to pass.

● *Insufficient knowledge or skills* – this often occurs due to a poor initial interview which has not identified the student's previous experience and has failed to identify the appropriate learning opportunities the student requires. In addition, students need time to develop knowledge and practice new skills, so if expectations by the practice supervisor or assessor are unrealistic the student can be left feeling overwhelmed or inadequate, which will impact on their confidence.

● *Personal problems at home* – these can have a significant impact on a student's ability to fully engage with the learning opportunities in practice. This can be compounded if they are not used to shift work.

So when faced with an underperforming student it is important not to immediately decide that it is the student's fault. Consider instead the influence that you as a practice supervisor/assessor can have in helping the student achieve their proficiencies or change their behaviour to achieve the required professional values.

When Does Underperformance Occur?

There is no one point during a student's placement where concerns should be identified about their performance. Each time a student is on duty is an opportunity to identify what the student is doing well and to reflect on whether the student's performance is enabling them to achieve the professional values and proficiencies set out in their PAD. Some students may initially be judged to be failing to achieve the required standard of proficiency during the early part of their placement. This could be because they take time to settle into a new environment. However, their performance may improve following feedback and the development of an action plan (if needed) and the end result is a pass. Other students may fail to reach the required level of proficiency or demonstrate the required professional values during their placement despite appropriate interventions, with the end result that they are recorded as failing to achieve one or more proficiencies or professional values. Whichever is the case, failing to achieve the expected standard at any stage during a placement means that the student is underperforming and may not pass at the final interview.

There is a potential third scenario, and that is the student who has not been identified as underperforming at the mid-point interview but is then found not to have met the required level of proficiency or met the professional values at the end point of the placement. This is a common occurrence and can occur for a number of reasons:

● failure by the practice supervisor/assessor to sufficiently monitor, assess and provide feedback across the length of the placement
● initial or mid-point interviews held too late (or not provided at all)
● the practice assessor 'hoping' that a student will improve given more time, without putting in place appropriate actions to support the student to succeed.

If there are concerns regarding a student's knowledge, skills or attitudes related to any assessment element during a placement, then alarm bells should start ringing. This will be the first warning sign that there may be a potential problem and should never be ignored. Hoping that a problem will just go away, or if the student is given more time they will improve, will never be the solution if no support is put in place. Actions must be taken as soon as a concern with a student's proficiency or professional behaviour becomes apparent.

If the initial interview was not conducted early enough, then the practice supervisor and assessor, and the student will not have identified what the student needed to achieve on their placement. As a consequence, it may take some time before the alarm bells really start ringing. Equally, failure to undertake the mid-point interview at the right time will also delay the opportunity to identify concerns. If concerns are identified without a well-documented initial interview more time will need to be spent reviewing the PAD to identify the specific proficiencies or professional values that link to the skills, knowledge or values causing concerns. If a student is not making the expected progress, then they need help and it is part of both the practice supervisor and the practice assessor's role to provide this support.

Practice Scenario

Jane is the practice assessor for Peter, a first-year child field student. Jane works in a children's day treatment centre where there is a high turnover of children every day and staff are constantly busy. Jane is concerned about Peter's communication skills with the parents of the children they are treating. He lacks confidence when speaking to the parents and avoids eye contact with them. Some parents have commented on his lack of engagement with them. Jane did not get a chance to look at Peter's proficiencies during the initial interview and it is the third week of Peter's placement before she looks at the PAD during the midpoint interview. To her horror, she realises that there is a specific proficiency that requires her to assess Peter's confidence in communicating with children and parents. Jane realises that Peter is currently not demonstrating the skills required to evidence achievement of this proficiency, but the placement is now halfway through and valuable time has been lost. Jane finds herself having to tell Peter that he is not meeting the requirements for this proficiency with very little time left to improve. She feels guilty and also angry that her manager has made her support students when the unit is so busy.

IDENTIFYING THE CONCERN

The first step to take when it is believed that a student is underperforming is to ascertain exactly what the concern is. Sometimes it is a very specific area of practice (poor time keeping, lack of knowledge regarding key medicines used in the placement). In some cases, however, staff use more general terms which can be more problematic in linking to a specific proficiency or professional value.

Common Causes of Concern

Duffy and Hardicre (2007) identified a number of common signs that may indicate a cause for concern about a student's performance which are listed below.

- Lack of interest and motivation.
- Inconsistency in achieving the required level of competence.
- Inconsistent clinical performance.
- Lack of insight into own weaknesses.
- Not responding appropriately to feedback.
- Limited practical, interpersonal and communication skills.
- Lack of theoretical knowledge.
- Absence of professional boundaries and behaviours.
- Experiencing poor health, for example withdrawn, tired, listless.
- Unreliable, regularly late or absent.

There must be evidence related to the concern, not just a hunch or a feeling. In the clinical scenario earlier, Jane has concerns related to Peter's communication skills. This needs to be evidenced by examples where his communication had been unsatisfactory. In this case it was both his verbal and non-verbal communication, and evidence could be given related to specific examples of his poor communication with relatives as well as the feedback Jane had received from some of the parents. For example, he did not greet the parents when he approached the child in order to take the child's temperature, pulse and respirations. He did not explain what he was going to do to the parents or the child.

While a one-off event may be a very early warning of a problem with proficiency, it is rarely a good idea to base a decision on just one example. Providing feedback in this situation on how they may have taken a different approach is still important. If a student is underperforming in relation to a specific proficiency, then it is preferable that there are several examples of this to evidence the concerns being raised. However, if there is an aspect of poor practice that could lead to harm, then it is essential to act quickly to remedy the situation.

It is essential to be clear what it is that you are concerned about and which proficiency or professional value this relates to before addressing the issue with the student. This does not mean waiting for weeks before discussing any concerns; rather, it is important to decide very quickly if there really is a problem and if so, the exact nature of the concerns and the evidence to support them. Try to identify if the concern relates to a student's knowledge, skill or their attitude, and have examples of how the student has failed to demonstrate the expected level of proficiency in practice. Once again, a good initial interview should have provided a very clear benchmark on which to base any decisions.

It is also important to recognise that some students lack confidence and take time to settle in, so do not make judgements too early. Early actions to support the student, however, are essential. It is also important to check whether a student has any reasonable adjustments that need to be put in place (see Chapter 10), as without the required reasonable adjustments the student may be unable to make the progress expected.

! If there are any concerns regarding a student's performance then make a quick note of the event that took place, the time and date, so that you can refer to this accurately when meeting with the student.

Ensuring Objectivity

The NMC requires that any assessment decision must be based on evidence and be objective and fair. Evidence from a range of sources ensures greater objectivity and cannot then be seen as a personal view. It is important, therefore, to consult with colleagues to gain their judgements of a student's progress, particularly if there are concerns regarding their performance. While one person's opinion could be subjective, a number of different viewpoints will dramatically increase the objectivity of an assessment decision. This is referred to as inter-assessor reliability. Ask the practice supervisors or other colleagues about their experience of working with the student to identify whether they have the same concerns. If no one else has noticed a problem, then it may be that the expectations are of a higher standard than is required for the student at their particular stage on the programme and there is a need to adjust those expectations. Alternatively, consider asking another practice assessor or the student's practice supervisor to spend time with the student to undertake their own assessment of the student in the areas of concern. If others are equally concerned regarding a student's performance, then this is the time to discuss the concerns with your student.

> ! Evidence from multiple sources ensures a fair and objective assessment.

DISCUSSING UNDERPERFORMANCE WITH STUDENTS

Once it has been determined that there is a particular area in which a student is failing to reach the expected level of proficiency it is essential to address this as soon as possible with them.

- The first step is to ask the student how they believe they are doing in relation to the aspect of performance that is causing concerns. An insightful student may identify their own concerns about the same areas that have been identified by the practice supervisor/assessor. If they do this, it will make it easier to then go on to discuss how this will be managed and they will be supported. Unfortunately, it is possible that they will say all is well. In this situation it will then be necessary to talk about the concerns that have been identified.
- Identify what the concern is.
- Provide the student with evidence of the concerns. This should be based on identifiable situations or events that have taken place during the placement that support the concerns and should be related to their knowledge, skill and/or attitude; they should be linked to the relevant proficiency or professional value. The evidence should be conclusive without being overwhelming. Ideally, this should include some instances where the person involved in giving the feedback was involved. If the practice supervisors or other staff have expressed concerns, ensure that the student is aware that others are equally concerned and that this is not one opinion. If the gathering of information from multiple sources was discussed at the initial interview, then this information should not provoke conflict.
- Be considerate of the student's feelings in the approach used when discussing the concerns.
- Be honest. If there is a problem, then the student must be very clear what it is, as they will need to know exactly in what way(s) they are not achieving the criteria for the specific proficiency or professional value before they can take steps to improve.

- Identify areas where the student is also doing well.
- Reinforce that support will be provided to help the student to improve.

Chapter 7 discussed feedback in depth, so refer to the advice provided in that chapter when providing feedback on concerns with a student.

Students Who Deny There Is a Problem

One of the more difficult aspects of supporting an underperforming student occurs when the student denies that there is a problem with their performance. In this situation there are two possible explanations.

1. The judgement made is incorrect – there are no problems with the student's performance and the evidence used to support the judgement made is inaccurate. This will require honest acknowledgement by the practice assessor and may require some further work to maintain the student's confidence in their judgement.
2. The judgement made is correct – there are problems with the student's performance, but the student is struggling to accept or acknowledge this. This is where evidence can assist the student in recognising that they are not making the required progress.

Coercive Strategies Used by Students

It is not unusual to meet students who find it difficult to accept that they are not achieving the performance standards set. Failing a pre-registration nursing course is high stakes for a student, as they are not only losing the opportunity to achieve their degree but also losing a future career. It is not unusual therefore to find a student who adopts a defensive stance, and significant pressure can be applied by the student on the practice assessor to pass them. Hunt et al. (2016) undertook a study which identified that some students used manipulative behaviours to try and coerce their mentors (this was prior to the SSSA standards) to change their decision. These coercive behaviours can have an impact on the assessor, causing guilt and fear. Four types of coercive students were identified:

- *Initiators* – students with likeable personalities, who are charming, obliging and emotionally exploitative. If told they are at risk of not passing, they might beg or cry. They cause a very high level of guilt because they are 'a nice person'.
- *Diverters* – students who use what are often irrelevant factors such as personal circumstances, illness or disability that are not relevant or applicable to the situation in an attempt to divert the focus away from their underperformance. They can cause a high level of guilt and anxiety.
- *Disparagers* – students who challenge the decision by belittling and denigrating in ways that may be perceived as professionally damaging to the

practice assessor by using terms such as *bullying* or *discriminatory*. This can cause a high level of fear.

- *Aggressors* – students who are openly hostile and may directly threaten the mentor verbally or physically. Such threats may come from third parties, such as friends or family members. This can cause a very high level of fear.

It is important to note that these behaviours are not commonplace, but to recognise that some students may use coercive behaviours when they believe they may be failed. It is essential to confirm whether the assessment process has been followed. This means that the decisions made were evidenced-based, objective and fair, and that appropriate support and appropriate learning opportunities were provided, with regular feedback to enable the student to improve their performance. If this is the case, then the responsibility for failing to achieve the required standard of performance lies with the student and not the practice supervisor or assessor. Where students use coercive behaviours, additional support may be needed, which will be looked at later in this chapter.

UNDERPERFORMANCE DOES NOT MEAN FAILURE

If a student is struggling to make the progress expected during their placement then it is very important they understand that that this does not mean they will fail at the end of the placement. Underperformance during the placement means that the required standard is not currently being reached; however, a final decision has not been made and there is time to improve.

Failing the placement can only happen at the end of the placement and is the result of failure to achieve the required standard in one or more proficiencies or professional values by the end of the placement. This is another reason to raise concerns early with a student. An early warning that improvements are required provides maximum opportunity to improve and decreases the possibility of end failure. Raising concerns late in the placements limits opportunities to improve, creates significant anxiety for the student and makes failure to succeed more likely.

> ! Alert the student as soon as possible if there are any concerns regarding their performance. This will give time to agree the appropriate actions and support to enable improvements to be made.

SUPPORTING UNDERPERFORMING STUDENTS

While raising concerns with a student regarding their performance in practice is an important part of the role of both supervisors and assessors, the responsibility does not end there. Having raised the concern, the next step is offering help and support to enable the student to improve in the areas identified. This will require dedicated time to provide the necessary ongoing support with regular feedback.

The act of offering help and support when identifying problems with students also lessens the emotional impact of the feedback they receive. If a student is given clear feedback along with a plan for support, then they will be far more willing to accept the assessment judgement. By exploring with the student how they can be helped, they will also be more willing to accept that there is a problem that needs resolving and engage in the process to make improvements.

Additional Support for the Underperforming Student

If the student is failing to achieve the required standard of proficiency or professional values, it is important to seek additional help. Requesting help at this stage will ensure the best decisions are made for the student and both the practice assessor and student feel supported through this process.

Support From Colleagues

The most obvious and immediate support available will be from colleagues within the practice area. There may be a number of people available to help including:

- the practice supervisor(s) who have been supporting the student
- more experienced practice assessors
- unit managers
- practice educators
- leads for practice education.

The decision to contact someone for support will in part be down to the experience of the practice assessor. There may be local policies or agreements as to who should be informed or called upon for support where concerns have been raised regarding a student's performance. The main point is that help is sought early in the assessment process. An underperforming student will require additional time in order to agree the action plan, implement it and provide the extra supervision, support and feedback they will require. This may require understanding colleagues at work who may need to help cover some of the day-to-day workload to give the practice supervisor and assessor the dedicated time needed to support the student. It is an expectation by the NMC that practice assessors have *supported time and resources to enable them to fulfil their roles* (NMC, 2018e), which in this situation may be additional time to support the student and the additional support of colleagues to achieve this.

University Support and the Role of the Academic Assessor

It is important to inform the university as soon as possible when a student is not making the expected progress. This ensures that support measures can be put in place for both the staff in practice and the student. If a student is failing to reach the required standard, then the practice supervisor, practice assessor *and* the student will need support. The key person available to help the practice assessor and the student is the student's academic assessor. In addition, the following people may also be able to provide support to the practice supervisor and assessor and/or the student:

- Link Lecturers
- lecturer practitioners
- programme leaders
- personal tutors.

Most universities have a dedicated practice team so they will also be available to support staff with underperforming students, and also support the students during this time.

DEVELOPING ACTION PLANS

The best way to ensure the appropriate support is provided is to involve the student in the development of an action plan. This should clearly indicate the aspects of their practice that require improvement and include the actions that will be taken to support the student. They should be involved in the development of the action plan as much as possible as they need to take ownership of the concerns identified, and the actions agreed. The focus should not be on the problem; rather, it should be on what they can do about it with support from their practice supervisor and practice assessor. Action plans should always be developed using the SMART acronym to ensure that everyone involved is clear what has been agreed and what the student is expected to demonstrate; this should include the date on which it is agreed. The SMART acronym stands for:

Specific	States what the student is expected to achieve in terms of knowledge, skills, and attitudes.
Measurable	Observable and assessable: clearly state the behaviour the student will demonstrate to show that they have achieved the outcome required.
Achievable	Within the student's range of abilities and available in their practice area
Realistic	Appropriate to the knowledge and skill level expected of the student.
Time scaled	Clear target dates set for achievement.

The important features of an action plan are a clearly identified problem or concern, a clear indication of what needs to be improved on and how this can be achieved, with examples of the support that will be provided. However, the most important element is agreeing what the student will need to demonstrate in order to show that they have achieved the required standard of competence. If the action plan is unclear on what they need to do, it will be very difficult to determine whether they have achieved it (Table 8.1). The action plan will

TABLE 8.1 An Example of an Action Plan

Nature of concern (link to proficiency or PVs)	What does the student need to demonstrate? (use SMART)	Support available & who is responsible	Reviews/ feedback
27/05/20 Bev finds it difficult to prioritise care needs and delegate care activities when caring for a group of service users (SUs). This leads to SUs not being ready for planned activities, observations not being recorded on time and documentation not completed by the end of the shift. (Proficiency 19)	When allocated a group of service users Bev needs to identify priorities for the shift and identify which care activities can be delegated and why. She will delegate appropriate care activities and check progress by her colleagues using clear communication. All documentation will be completed as care is completed and fully completed 30 min before the end of the shift.	Bev will be allocated a group of service users each shift and her practice supervisor and assessor will be given protected time to ensure she is supported on each shift. A reflective discussion will be undertaken each day with Bev to identify progress and areas to focus on for the next shift. Dates for review: 01/06/20 & 08/06/20	01.06.20 Bev has been allocated a group of service users each shift & is using time at the start of each day to identify priorities & making brief notes to keep on track – this aspect is much improved. Bev continues to try and do most of the work herself. We have discussed reasons for not delegating and strategies she can use to approach staff and request help. We will focus on this for the next three shifts and review again. 6/6/20

provide an additional benchmark that can be referred to as evidence of continued development and demonstrates evidence that the assessment process is being followed. A documented action plan also provides evidence that the practice assessor is fulfilling their professional accountability and responsibility, by identifying learning needs, facilitating learning opportunities and undertaking a fair and evidence-based assessment.

> ! Action plans provide evidence that the assessment process is being followed if a student is not meeting the progress expected and can ensure support is identified to help the student to improve.

THE IMPORTANCE OF CLEAR DOCUMENTATION

Throughout the student's placement there should be clear and accurate records maintained in the student's assessment documentation of their progress and any areas of concern. There will be formal records at the initial, midpoint and final interview, which this book covers. However, additional records should also be maintained for significant events throughout a student's placement. Clearly written records of any feedback and actions agreed must be included in the student's PAD, including any action plans. The types of information that should be recorded are:

- areas of good practice demonstrated by the student
- specific professional values or proficiencies that are of concern
- reasons and evidence of concern
- summary of feedback and discussions with student
- help provided, dates, people involved, etc.
- documented action plans.

Make sure all documentation is factual and ensure the student feels a part of the action plan to help them commit to achieving success. Consistent and honest feedback will be essential. If improvement is being made, then make sure the student is aware of this and document what improvements have been seen. If improvements are not being made, then also ensure that the student is informed and it is documented. Try not to overload the student with too much feedback and ensure positive areas of practice are identified.

It is important to remember that external examiners from other universities are required to review students' assessments to ensure that the university assessment processes and decisions are fair. This includes reviewing a sample of PADs each year, so what is written in a PAD may be subject to external scrutiny.

SERIOUS CONCERNS

If a student's practice or behaviour raises serious concerns or there are patient/service user safety risks due to poor practice or behaviours, the academic assessor and university must be contacted immediately. If there is fitness-to-practice concern, then the university will need to implement their fitness-to-practice process. Where there is an immediate risk to patients/service users or staff or the concerns relate to the student's own well-being, then the student's placement may need to be stopped immediately pending a discussion with the academic assessor or senior member of staff from the university.

Ensure all concerns in this situation are well-documented with dates and times and the people involved. Keep details factual with what happened and what was said. This will form the basis for evidence that may be required if a decision is made that the student needs to be referred to a fitness-to-practice panel at the university. If the student is an apprentice or a secondee then their employer will need to be informed as well.

MAKING THE FINAL ASSESSMENT DECISION

Planned support provided to an underperforming student during a placement which is well-documented is important for three reasons.

1. A student who is not making the expected progress can improve if the support provided focusses on the identified areas for improvement.
2. Well-documented decisions, based on evidence, with SMART action plans where required, will ensure that due process has been followed and the assessment process is valid.
3. Evidence of following the assessment process and providing the right support to the student acts as evidence that practice supervisors and practice assessors have fulfilled their responsibility as required by the NMC *Code* and the NMC SSSA (2018b).

Unfortunately, despite support and regular feedback some students will not reach the required standard of proficiency in all the required areas by the end of the placement and therefore cannot be signed-off as having achieved the required proficiencies or professional values and so will not meet the requirements for a pass. The final assessment decision will therefore be to record 'not achieved' against the relevant assessment elements. However, it is acknowledged that informing a student they have not met the criteria for a pass is difficult.

When a student submits their theory assignment there will be a delay before the results are officially released to the student and they normally read them online. However, practice assessments are very different; the student will know the outcome immediately. If a student has not passed any of the elements in their practice assessment, then they will know the decision immediately at the final interview. They also know the practice assessor who has made that decision. Unlike theoretical assessments, the practice assessment decision is made face to face and so it becomes especially difficult for both the student and the practice assessor, especially if they have formed a positive relationship with each other. Where there is face-to-face feedback there may be the added potential for conflict if there is disagreement about the assessment decision. The accuracy and reliability of feedback that has been provided throughout the placement will then be especially important to support the decision.

! If it is a student's first attempt, rather than tell them that they have failed their assessment, tell them that they have not met the criteria for a pass.

Feeling Guilty

Many practice assessors feel guilty when they have to tell a student they have not passed their assessment. Professional relationships and caring behaviours are an important part of being a nurse and failing a student can be seen as uncaring. As a consequence, the practice assessor may 'fail to fail' the student at the end of their placement.

FAILING TO FAIL

Failing to fail describes the situation where a student who is not making the expected progress is still passed at the end of their placement. It is unclear how many students are actually failed in practice. A study by Hunt et al. (2012) found that very few students in the UK failed their practice assessment in comparison with the numbers who failed their theoretical assessments, but North et al. (2019) argue that this does not necessarily mean that staff in practice fail to fail students. Assessment in practice is far more complex, making many assessment decisions less clear cut than is seen with an academic assessment. Also assessment in practice is continuous, providing students with feedback when they are not making the required progress and therefore given time to make the required improvement. If completed essays were submitted for feedback, following which students made the required corrections and then submitted for marking, then failure at the first attempt at academic assessments would fall significantly!

North et al. (2019) describe the psychological and emotional impact of failing a student. Guilt is common amongst practice supervisors and assessors if their student is not successful in practice. The process of informing a student they will not pass their placement can be stressful, especially if they feel unable to access appropriate support within their workplace or from the university. These feelings can lead the practice assessor to give the student the benefit of the doubt and pass the student in the hope that the student will improve on their next placement. This is more likely to occur in year one and year two of a student's programme. Some of the more common reasons for failing to fail include:

- Failure to establish the evidence to achieve the criteria for each proficiency. The practice assessor may fail to fail if they are unsure what standard of proficiency the student is required to demonstrate. Under these circumstances they pass students who have 'worked hard' or 'shown enthusiasm'.
- Failure to consistently assess a student's performance throughout the placement. Practice assessors may fail to fail because they did not observe the student's performance and there is limited evidence from practice supervisors on which to base their final assessment. This situation can easily arise if the practice supervisor and practice assessor are not rostered to work alongside the student frequently enough.

- Failure to highlight concerns with a student about their poor performance on placement. Practice assessors may fail to fail if they do not raise their concerns regarding a student's performance. This situation often arises when the practice assessor hopes that the student will improve without the need to raise concerns and inform the university. If the student has not been informed of concerns throughout the placement there is a high likelihood of conflict at the end if they are then told they have failed. The practice assessor may then fail to fail in order to avoid potential conflict.
- Failure to fail also happens when the assessment process has not been followed. This includes lack of/or insufficient feedback, a delayed or even no midpoint interview which leads the practice assessor to avoid conflict with their student at the final assessment.
- Failure to understand their professional accountability and responsibility. This can occur when staff have not been appropriately prepared for their role and do not appreciate the significance of passing a student who is not making the required progress.

An appreciation of the impact of passing a student who has not met the required level of proficiency on previous placement often only occurs when the student has progressed to the end of their programme. At that point a practice assessor is faced with assessing a student who has consistently underperformed but never been informed of this and is shocked when told on their last placement that they will not pass. It is at this point, where a practice assessor is required to sign off a student who will go on to the NMC register, that a realisation of accountability occurs. Students are more likely to be failed on their final placement than their first one.

Failing Can Be a Positive Action

If a student is underperforming and not meeting the required level of proficiency, not passing them can be a positive. By not doing this a student has been denied the access to the help and support they need. On their next placement an assumption will be made that they have met the required level of proficiency, and the student will be expected to build on that. The student will be left struggling with no plan or process for improving the areas they need to develop.

Informing a student that they have not passed is a professional (not a personal) decision based on evidence and demonstrates an understanding of the accountability and responsibility that comes with the role. By identifying an underperforming student, action plans will have been developed, support will be made available and the student can be supported to achieve. Even if they do not pass at the end of the placement the next practice supervisor and assessor will be aware that the student needs support and from day one can put in the appropriate level of support the student requires. This provides the student with every opportunity to improve in a different practice environment and potentially succeed.

The Importance of the Ongoing Achievement Record

The reasons as to why a student has failed to make the progress required to pass a placement must also be documented in their ongoing achievement record (OAR). This is not only a summary of the events that took place on the placement; it is also the opportunity to inform the next practice supervisor and practice assessor about the support the student requires. The more detailed the information provided about any specific concerns and the support the student will require, the more help the next practice supervisors and assessors can provide. Often practice assessors will sanitise what they say, not wishing to leave negative comments in the student's OAR or be viewed as uncaring. This again denies the student help and support from the start of their next placement, which is not a kindness.

> ! When completing the ongoing achievement record try to put yourself in the next practice assessor's shoes. What information will they find most useful, what advice would you give them? Write the information that you would like to receive.

WHAT HAPPENS WHEN A STUDENT IS NOT SUCCESSFUL?

There are some misguided beliefs about the impact of not passing a student. Many students and staff in practice believe that if a student is not passed at the end of their placement then the following consequences may occur:

- the student's career prospects are ruined
- the student will be discontinued from the programme
- the placement will gain a reputation for having 'hard' practice assessors
- the placement will gain a reputation for being uncaring towards students.

Fortunately none of these consequences are accurate. They are, however, popular myths that many students and practice staff worry about despite no supportive evidence. Failing to pass a student does not result in ruining a student's career or having them discontinued from their course if it is their first attempt at practice. Rather it leads to the opportunity for a second attempt at the elements within the practice assessment document that they failed to achieve.

Second Attempts

It is the norm in most universities that a student is automatically granted a second attempt if they have not passed their assessment at the first attempt, and this follows for the practice element of the programme. If a student does not pass, this should not come as a surprise to the university as they should already be aware of this possibility through contact with the Link Lecturer and academic assessor. When the assessment document is handed in to the university then the assessment result will be recorded as a fail at first attempt (or as a 'refer') and the student will be offered a second attempt. The second attempt may be repeated on the same placement or may be held in a different clinical area to the first attempt to allow for new practice supervisors and assessors to assess the student's performance.

Supporting Students on a Second Attempt at Practice

Supporting a student who is undertaking a second attempt at practice can be quite challenging, as the student may enter the placement with low self-esteem or feeling very anxious and worried. The role of both the practice supervisor and practice assessor will still be to provide a range of learning opportunities with a focus on the elements that have not been passed and provide a fair and objective assessment. All the advice given in earlier chapters around planning learning opportunities and the assessment process apply. To recap, these are:

- undertake the initial interview as soon as possible in the first week
- look at the feedback in the PAD from the previous placement where the student failed at the first attempt and at the comments in the ongoing achievement record
- identify the assessment elements that need to be re-assessed and agree an action plan with SMART objectives to help the student achieve the required elements
- schedule regular meetings to review progress and provide honest feedback on their performance
- if the student is not making the progress required seek help from the Link Lecturer or academic assessor from the university.

Clear and consistent feedback is probably one of the most essential elements as the student will need to be informed of their progress and to be informed early on if they are not making the required progress. As the second attempt is a student's opportunity to demonstrate that they have developed and improved on the first attempt there should be very clear expectations of what the student needs to demonstrate in order to achieve the assessment elements they did not pass at the first attempt. The content and accuracy of the ongoing achievement record will be invaluable for providing the basis on which to plan the support the student needs.

First and Second Attempts Together

Sometimes students may be required to undertake their second attempt at the assessment elements they did not pass and at the same time be required to undertake new assessments on their new placement. This will usually happen when only a small number of assessment elements are outstanding, and it is not in the student's interest to prevent their progression and will depend on the policies at the university. If supporting a student who only needs to undertake a second attempt on the elements they did not pass before, it is important to remember that these must be the main focus, although there is an expectation that they continue to demonstrate the required professional values as well.

If a student is required to be assessed for a second attempt on elements from a previous placement and is also undertaking first attempts on new elements still to be achieved in their PAD, this means being very organised in supporting the student. This is even more true if they have two PADs, having commenced the next part of their programme. However, the ongoing achievement record will act as a reference point for what the focus is for the placement. Reflecting on the feedback in the ongoing achievement record with the student will help the development of the action plans for the placement.

> ! Discuss the student's action plan with colleagues so they can support the student if there are times when their practice supervisor/assessor is not available.

When the student has two PADS the skills of planning for and facilitating learning will be necessary. It is advisable to undertake an initial, midpoint and final interview for each set of assessment elements. This will help distinguish what is required for each assessment, and though a little more documentation is involved it will enable the student to focus on what needs to be done for first and second attempts. The ongoing achievement record should also be completed after a second attempt, regardless of the outcome.

THE FINAL ASSESSMENT DECISION

The final assessment decision should never come as a surprise to the student. Throughout their placement the student should have received regular feedback on their progress and so they should have an indication of what the final outcome will be. As long as due process has been followed with documented evidence of a clear action plan with regular feedback, if the student has still been unable to achieve the required level of proficiency at the required assessment elements or demonstrated the required professional values then the final decision has to be to fail the student. Always seek support from the university in this situation. This will be a difficult interview to undertake and so having the academic assessor or Link Lecturer present at the final assessment will provide support to both the practice assessor and the student. Afterwards it may be helpful to discuss the whole process with the Link Lecturer to gain reassurance that the assessment process was followed, and no opportunities were missed.

REFLECTING ON THE EXPERIENCE OF SUPPORTING AN UNDERPERFORMING STUDENT

It is not unusual for a practice assessor to feel that failing a student at the second attempt reflects badly on them. They fear being labelled as unkind, harsh or unfair. However, it is important to understand that if the assessment process has been evidence-based, fair and objective then there are justified reasons for the student not passing.

It is good practice after supporting a student for a practice assessor to reflect on their own performance. Instead of being focused on the result the student achieved, they should assess their own performance. The following checklist can be used to assess your own performance and keep the outcomes for your next revalidation review meeting. For any questions where the answer is *no*, consider why that is.

- Did I review feedback on the student's previous placement and agree clear goals and objectives at the initial interview?
- Did I check whether the student required any reasonable adjustments to support them to achieve the requirements of the proficiencies or professional values?
- Did I make sufficient opportunities to observe the student in practice?
- Did I inform my student as early as possible of concerns related to their performance?
- Did I discuss with the student the support they required?
- Did we develop an action plan together?
- Did I provide feedback and discuss this with the student and check their understanding?
- Did I provide a timely midpoint interview?
- Did I document concerns, support and advice throughout the placement?
- Did I get help and support from my colleagues and the university?
- Did my student reach the required standard and if so, how did I contribute to that success?
- Did I fail my student and if so, reflecting on their time on placement is there anything I could have done differently?

Reflecting on both positive and less positive experiences of supporting students contributes to a registered nurse's personal development and is a requirement of the NMC's revalidation process (NMC, 2019a). Requesting feedback from colleagues and the university after supporting a student through a re-assessment can provide another perspective and gives alternative views that may not have been considered. As a registered nurse it is important to remember that the NMC (2018f) requires practice assessors to:

- Take responsibility for carrying out a reliable and evidenced-based assessment, including all assessment decisions.

● Take action to ensure any concerns raised with the student are dealt with in a timely and appropriate manner.

Following this guidance ensures that whatever the outcome may be, the assessment process has been duly followed.

Action Points

1. Take time to read the practice assessment documents used by your local universities to ensure you are familiar with what the students are required to achieve.
2. Seek guidance from the university for any elements within the PAD that you are unsure of.
3. Find out what the process is for raising concerns regarding a student's fitness to practice.

Chapter 9

Confirming Achievement

Chapter Outline

INTRODUCTION

The purpose of this chapter is to explore the nature and function of the final interview and the confirming of achievement by the practice assessor. The final interview is the event that takes place at the end of each placement. The essential components of a successful final interview will be identified and the process for conducting it, ensuring that the process confirms a valid assessment and confirmation of a student's achievement in practice learning or clearly documents that a student has not met the criteria for a pass.

A Nurse's Survival Guide to Supervising and Assessing. https://doi.org/10.1016/B978-0-7020-8147-7.00009-0

The practice assessor and the academic assessor both have roles in confirming achievement; the practice assessor confirms achievement related to the student's learning in practice and the academic assessor confirms achievement in the university. It is the responsibility of the university in partnership with their practice partners to ensure that a student does not progress from one part of the programme to the next or progress at the end of their programme to enter the register if they have not met the required standards set out in the NMC's (2018d) *Standards of proficiency for registered nurses.* Therefore, at the end of each part of a student's programme, recommendation for progression is also made in partnership between the practice assessor and the academic assessor.

CONFIRMING ACHIEVEMENT

Confirmation of achievement is a requirement at key points in a student's programme. For practice learning it will take place at the end of each placement at the end of each part. When the practice assessor confirms a student's achievement, they are stating that they are satisfied that the student has achieved the required proficiencies and programme outcomes that they have been assessed on. This relates to the period of time that the practice assessor was assigned to the student and in doing so they are confirming that the assessment process was evidenced based, fair and objective.

The Practice Assessor's Responsibility for Confirming Achievement

The practice assessor is responsible for confirming a student's achievement of learning in practice. This will usually be for a single placement; however, a practice assessor can be responsible for assessing and confirming a student's achievement across more than one placement if they are in the same part (or year) of a student's programme.

The NMC *Standards* (2018b,e) set out a number of expectations and requirements of the practice assessor in fulfilling this role.

1. They should have an understanding of the student's previous and current achievement in practice and in theory.
2. They should have opportunities to observe the student in practice during the period assigned.
3. During the period the practice assessor is allocated to the student, the assessment of the student should be a continuous process with the practice assessor seeking and/or collating feedback from other sources on the student's progress; i.e. it is not a one-off event!
4. They should have opportunity to provide feedback to the student during their period of practice learning (through informal and formal meetings).

5. They should ensure that the assessment process is evidence based, fair and objective (see Chapter 7).
6. They must hand over to the next practice assessor (unless it is the final placement of the programme). The format for this is not prescribed and in most cases will be through completion of the practice assessment document (PAD) and ongoing achievement record (OAR) which should include identification of the student's strengths and areas for development.
7. If there are concerns about a student who is not meeting the progress expected, then they should inform the academic assessor and work with them and/or the Link Lecturer to develop action plans to support the student to improve (see Chapter 8).

The Academic Assessor's Responsibility for Confirming Achievement

The academic assessor is responsible for confirming student achievement within the academic environment (university). Usually there is one academic assessor for each part of the student's programme. A student cannot have the same academic assessor for two consecutive parts of a programme (but they could have the same academic assessor for parts one and three of a programme). For short programmes such as prescribing programmes or return to practice where there is only one part to the programme, the student will have one practice assessor and one academic assessor.

The NMC *Standards* (2018b,e) set out a number of expectations and requirements of the academic assessor in fulfilling this role.

1. They should have an understanding of the student's previous and current achievement in practice and in theory.
2. The collection and collation of the student's progress and achievement in their academic assessments should be continuous over the period that the academic assessor is allocated to the student. The NMC (2018f) suggest the following evidence may be used:
   - Student documentation, e.g. practice assessment document or the ongoing record of achievement, assessment records;
   - Academic course work and assessments;
   - Communication with staff delivering and assessing academic assignments and exams in the programme, if relevant;
   - Communication with the practice assessor(s);
   - Student self-reflections;
   - Communication and an ongoing relationship with the student;
   - Communication with anyone else who may be involved in the education of the student, for example course leader, personal tutor.

3. There should be communication with the practice assessor at the relevant points in the student's programme; the process for this will have been agreed between practice partners and the university.
4. They must ensure accurate record keeping of the student's achievements and progress.
5. They should hand over to the next academic assessor (unless it is the end of the programme).
6. If there are concerns with a student who is not meeting the progress expected in practice, then they will work with the practice assessor and the student to improve the student's performance e.g. development of action plans (see Chapter 8).
7. Where there are serious concerns regarding the student's conduct and/or performance they may, after discussion with the practice assessor, make the decision to withdraw the student from practice. This may include a referral to the university Fitness to Practice panel.

It can be seen from the above that the roles of the practice assessor and academic assessor are complimentary and require communication between them both. The way that they communicate and work together will have been agreed by the university and their practice partners and may include regular meetings together at key points with the student, or communication by phone, email, on-line or through documentation in the practice assessment document (PAD) and ongoing achievement record (OAR).

Protection of the Public

The development of the roles of academic and practice assessor by the NMC was to ensure protection of the public. This includes:

- ensuring that the assessments that are carried out are evidenced based, objective and fair
- raising concerns regarding the student's conduct or performance if appropriate
- acting promptly if any concerns are raised
- acting as role models in demonstrating safe and effective practice.

Both practice assessors and academic assessors also have a responsibility to abide by the duty of candour (NMC & General Medical Council, 2015). This also applies in their feedback to the student and means they must be open and honest with the student if they are not meeting the progress required, in theory or in practice and agree actions and support to enable the student to improve their performance.

RECOMMENDING A STUDENT FOR PROGRESSION

Confirmation of progression takes place at the end of each part of the programme. The practice assessor and the academic assessor work in partnership in recommending a student for progression. In making the recommendation they are expected to consider the student's performance in both theory and practice across the whole part of the programme. For the practice assessor who has only supported the student on the final placement for the part of the programme that they are on, this requires them to:

- Review the student's progress on previous placements, checking that the student has passed all the required assessment elements in the PAD for that part of the programme.
- Review the student's achievements on previous parts of the programme (i.e. if the student is on part 2 or part 3 of the programme) to assure themselves that the student is making the expected progress through each part.
- Identify if concerns were raised regarding a student's performance in a previous part and these concerns remain in the current part. If so, then recommendation for progression may not be appropriate. In this situation the student should have been assessed as 'not achieved' on one or more professional values or proficiencies relevant to the concern identified.

The academic assessor will need to review the student's progress across all parts of the programme and where there are concerns regarding a student's academic performance may discuss with the student's personal tutor additional academic support the student requires to improve their performance at the university.

Again, the way that the practice assessor and academic assessor communicate to agree progression will have been agreed by the university and their practice partners and may include a meeting at the progression point with the student, or communication by phone, email, on-line or through the documentation in the PAD and OAR.

The progression decision also requires them to take into consideration the student's conduct and their demonstration of the professional values expected of them. Professional values are assessed within the PAD so are taken into account through the assessment process. In the university a student's conduct and professional values will be looked at in relation to their engagement with the programme or concerns that have been raised such as academic misconduct, a student's health and well-being or behaviours that raise concerns regarding a student's fitness to practice. Where concerns have been raised and a student's conduct has not improved or concerns remain then the relevant university processes may be invoked such as fitness to practice.

No Compensation

An additional responsibility for the two roles is their duty to ensure that 'no compensation' is made at the final assessment decision and for decisions on progression. Practice staff often comment on how well a student performs in practice and cannot understand why they may not be performing so well at university. Equally some students are academically strong but less proficient in practice. The NMC (2018f) emphasises that a student's *'good achievement in practice must not in any way mitigate poor achievement in the academic environment, and vice versa'*. Where a student is underperforming in practice, the fact that the student is doing well academically is not a reason to pass them in practice. Equally the university cannot pass a student academically just because the student has received excellent reports in practice. In both cases the student must demonstrate their proficiency in both theory and practice.

THE FINAL INTERVIEW

One of the last events to take place during a student's placement is the final interview. This will always be a significant event for the student. The practice assessor is required to undertake a final interview with the student and confirm that the student has met the assessment criteria, which are set out in the PAD, to enable them to confirm their proficiency in the required elements or to confirm that they have not met the required level of proficiency in one or more elements. The latter will result in the student being recorded as not having passed that placement.

The final interview and confirmation of achievement in practice should take place with a student in the last week of their placement, ideally on the penultimate or final day of the placement if possible. If the interview is undertaken too early there is the potential that the student's performance and motivation to learn will diminish. A final interview that takes place too early also negates the opportunity for continual assessment throughout the entire placement period; it's a bit like finishing a 100-metre race at the 80-metre mark.

The Aim of the Final Interview

The final interview is the final, formal stage of the assessment process for a student on a practice placement. During the final interview the practice assessor will have the opportunity to review the placement experience with the student and their progress in meeting the different assessment elements within the PAD. The final interview should not be used as an opportunity for one-off tests or quizzes. By the time the final interview has been reached the student should already be aware of how they have performed during the placement through ongoing feedback and should not receive any surprises regarding the final assessment decision.

The final interview also provides the practice assessor with the opportunity for confirming the final assessment decision of the student's performance on placement. This assessment decision should be drawn from the evidence provided through the continuous assessment process that has taken place over the entire placement, using feedback from multiple sources including feedback from the practice supervisors. It is an opportunity to provide summarised feedback to the student on their overall performance during the placement and guidance for the ongoing development of the student, whatever their stage on the programme. The aim is always to conduct an assessment that is evidence based, fair and objective, maintains a student's self-esteem and motivates them to continue to develop their knowledge, skills and professional values.

> ! The final interview must always include identifying the student's strengths and areas for further development. How this is managed can have a major impact on their self-esteem and motivation to continue to develop their knowledge and skills further.

Content of the Final Interview

You may find it useful to consider developing a final interview checklist that can be used to guide the discussion throughout the interview (if one is not already present in the PAD). Not only will this ensure that all areas are covered, it will also ensure that all documentation is completed and that no elements in the PAD are missed or forgotten. If an e-PAD is being used then it should show if you have missed anything on its dashboard or create an alert if any sections have not been completed.

However, having your own checklist can also help to keep the interview within the designated timeframe as this provides a fixed agenda that both the student and the practice assessor can use. Key elements to consider are listed below.

- Checking that the record of practice supervisors and practice assessors has been completed by the relevant staff with signatures.
- Checking an initial and mid-point interview has been completed.
- Checking all professional values and relevant proficiencies and episodes of care/in-placement assessments that have been assessed have been signed off (as achieved or not achieved as appropriate).
- Final feedback provided and recorded in relation to: professional values/ behaviour, learning proficiencies and any required episodes of care/in-place assessments that the student has undertaken during the placement.
- Final feedback completed on any action plans used.
- Feedback on the student's experiences on placement, including feedback on own performance.
- Debrief on significant events if not undertaken before.
- All areas requiring a signature have been completed.
- Completion or verification of placement hours and any other documentation required by the university.
- Completion of the ongoing achievement record if a separate document.

Final Feedback to the Student

The final interview should involve a summary of the placement as a whole. The ongoing feedback throughout the placement should have kept the student informed of their progress towards meeting their proficiencies which ideally have been signed off as they progressed through their placement rather than leaving them all to the end of the placement. The final interview should therefore be a discussion of the evidence of the student's overall performance, with a clear explanation of the reasons for the final assessment decision. If the student has demonstrated evidence of the required level of proficiency during the placement then this is an opportunity to discuss relevant examples and provide positive feedback to the student on their achievements. It is also an opportunity to provide guidance on any areas the student can develop for future practice experiences. If the student has not demonstrated evidence of the required level of proficiency in any of the elements in the PAD, then this will be reflected in the final assessment decision. The final interview will then be used to discuss why the student has not met the criteria for a pass and how they might develop the areas identified as 'not achieved' in future placements.

! Don't forget to use the feedback sandwich when delivering feedback at the end of the placement. Not only will this keep your conversation structured, it will also ensure that the feedback is balanced and maintains a student's self-esteem.

It is very important that the final assessment decision does not contain 'surprise' assessment decisions. The feedback a student receives at their final interview should not be new or unexpected information, nor should it come as a shock. Remember that the feedback at this event should be a summary of feedback from the entire placement, so elements of this feedback will have been given at different stages in the student's placement. If new information is provided at the final assessment that may indicate a student will not pass their placement then it suggests that there has been a failure in the assessment process. The decision at the final assessment should summarise feedback across the placement and identify areas where the student has demonstrated improvement and areas for further development.

Feedback on the Student's Experience on the Placement

The final interview should also provide the student with an opportunity to provide feedback on their experience on the placement. This may be difficult, as the student may feel unable to be honest given that an assessment decision is to be made. If questions are asked after the final assessment decision, then their response may be influenced by whether they were informed that they had passed or not. The reality is that gaining feedback is problematic as the student is vulnerable.

The questions therefore need to be broad enough that a student can be honest without fearing that their responses may influence the outcome of the assessment. For example:

- What three things did the staff do well on this placement that contributed to your learning?
- What areas could we improve upon to enhance the experience for future students?

Some students may feel awkward in providing feedback directly to their practice assessor especially if they believe it will affect their assessment outcome. If a good rapport has been developed between the student and the practice assessor during the placement then honest communication between the two should be possible. The willingness of a student to provide feedback is feedback in itself, as it demonstrates that they feel comfortable enough to do so.

It may be that student feedback sheds light on areas of practice that need to be addressed, either personally or related to the unit or department. For this reason, the feedback the student provides will be invaluable in developing the quality of supervision and assessment within the placement and ensuring that the practice environment is supportive of students.

Debrief on Significant Events

During any placement there will be events and circumstances that affect students in different ways. Whilst a debrief after a significant event in practice should take place as soon as possible after it occurs it can be helpful to discuss this again at the end of the placement when the student has had time to reflect on what happened. As novices in the clinical environment, students are not only learning the how and why of nursing but developing the coping mechanisms they will require throughout their careers which will help them to develop the resilience they will need as a registered nurse.

! If there have been particularly difficult experiences during the placement that have impacted on a student, then discuss this with the Link Lecturer or academic assessor from the university. This will ensure that the student receives ongoing care and support following the placement.

MAKING THE FINAL ASSESSMENT DECISION

Each university will have agreed with practice partners which elements in a PAD that the practice supervisor will be able to sign-off and which elements the practice assessor will be required to assess and sign-off. This will be stated in the guidance section in the PAD or shown in the dashboard for an e-PAD.

As discussed before, in most cases a practice assessor will usually only be assigned for one placement. Being assigned across more than one placement may occur where a placement does not have a suitably prepared practice assessor. For example, a GP practice only has one registered nurse who will act as the practice supervisor on the student's final placement in part 2 of their programme. The student therefore requires a registered nurse from another organisation to act as the practice assessor. In this situation it may be arranged that the practice assessor from the student's previous placement will also be the practice assessor for this next placement. The practice assessor will still need to have an opportunity to observe the student at the GP practice but would not need to be based there. They will make an assessment decision for that placement as a separate decision from the first placement the student had with them.

Evidence to Make the Assessment Decision

In Chapter 7 the importance of an assessment decision being evidence based, fair and objective was discussed in detail. At the point of the final interview the practice assessor will need to check that the assessment decisions within the PAD meet the three criteria above. Therefore, the practice assessor must have access to the PAD in advance of the final meeting in order that they can check the assessment is fair and reliable and based on documented evidence that is robust and that all required elements have been completed and any actions identified have been completed and outcomes recorded. The evidence will include feedback from practice supervisors, service user feedback and the student's own reflections.

If any evidence is deemed insufficient, unfair or unreliable then the practice assessor must take actions to ensure that the evidence is more robust prior to the final assessment decision. This may be through discussions with the practice supervisor(s) or they may decide to undertake further observation of the student in practice to gather the additional evidence that is required to ensure the assessment decision is fair and reliable.

It is very important that the student receives feedback on their whole performance during the placement. This feedback should be based on a wide range of learning experiences and provided by the practice supervisor(s) as well as the practice assessor. This is very different from the past when one mentor would undertake this role and ensure a fair and more objective assessment.

Discussing final assessment decisions with other practice supervisors and staff can improve the reliability of the assessment decision. While the final interview may be an opportunity to complete the assessment documentation, it should not be seen as an assessment in itself. The assessment of performance should have taken place throughout the entire length of the student's placement, it should have been continuous and the student should have received constant feedback regarding their progress towards achieving learning outcomes. While the practice supervisor(s) will have played a significant role in formulating learning experiences and contributed to the assessment of the student's performance, it is also likely that the student will have undertaken learning experiences with other staff throughout the placement. These experiences will all have contributed to the assessment of the student's performance. The role of the practice assessor therefore is to draw upon all this experience throughout the placement as evidence of progress of the learning that has taken place. Objectivity comes through an overview of many experiences, not just one individual's opinion or experience.

By the time the final interview is reached therefore there should be a range of documented evidence that will assist the practice assessor to finalise the assessment. As feedback during the student's placement should have been provided in both verbal and written form (or in the e-PAD) this should provide a good basis for discussion and finalising the paperwork.

Additional Evidence to Consider Within the PAD

In addition to evidence from practice supervisors, there should also be evidence of reflections by the student on their learning, the episodes of care/in-point assessments and practice experiences outside of the main placement.

Students are also required to seek feedback from service users. Whilst the tools used tend to be very simple and patients and service users rarely provide feedback that criticises the student's performance these should be looked at and discussed at the final interview alongside the student's own reflections.

Criteria for Assessment

The assessment document will require the practice assessor to confirm the student's achievement. The way the decision is to be recorded may vary according to the different types of assessment documentation, so it is important to understand how the PAD should be completed. No matter the format, the most important aspect is that the decision made is based on evidence of continuous assessment and is fair and reliable.

Each PAD will have the criteria against which the performance of the student should be assessed and these are helpful in clarifying the performance the student is expected to demonstrate. Over the three parts of the programme the student will demonstrate increasing independence and confidence. Examples of assessment criteria for the three parts of the programme are:

Part 1: Guided participation in care and performing with increasing confidence and competence.
Part 2: Active participation in care with minimal guidance and performing with increased confidence and competence.

Part 3: Practising independently with minimal supervision and leading and coordinating care with confidence (Pan London Practice Learning Group, 2019a).

Some countries have broken these overarching criteria down further to identify the skills, knowledge and professional values that the student must demonstrate to meet the criteria at each level. Box 9.1 shows examples of the assessment criteria used in England and Wales for a student in part 3 of their programme.

! If you need help in understanding the assessment criteria, then seek advice before the final interview.

DOCUMENTING THE ONGOING ACHIEVEMENT RECORD

At the end of a student's placement their ongoing achievement record must also be completed if it is a separate document. This should take the form of a summary of the student's strengths and areas for further development. This should reflect the evidence and feedback in the PAD and match all the information that was discussed with the student at the final interview.

BOX 9.1 Assessment Criteria for Part 3 of the Student's Programme

All Wales Practice Assessment Document and Ongoing Record of Achievement, 2020

	Knowledge	Skills	Professional values
Achieved	Is able to give a comprehensive account of the knowledge underpinning the proficiency	Confidently and proficiently demonstrates a range of appropriate skills to ensure safe person-centred care	Resilient and accountable for own actions and takes responsibility for own learning and that of others
	Pan London Practice Learning Group (2019a) – criteria used across England		
Achieved	Has a comprehensive knowledgebase to support safe and effective practice and can critically justify decisions and actions using an appropriate evidence base.	Is able to safely, confidently and competently manage person-centred care in both predictable and less well recognised situations, demonstrating appropriate evidence-based skills.	Acts as an accountable practitioner in responding proactively and flexibly to a range of situations. Takes responsibility for own learning and the learning of others.

The ongoing achievement record will be invaluable for the student and the practice supervisors and practice assessors on the next placement. They will be able to use the information contained in the ongoing achievement record to inform and develop learning plans for the next placement. If a student still needs to develop further competence in a particular proficiency or professional value, this can be documented and then they and their next practice supervisor and assessor will be provided with clear details regarding the areas that the student requires the most support in. Equally, recording evidence of their achievements means that they can plan new experiences that extend and consolidate proficiencies already achieved. Stretching a high-achieving student is equally as important as developing those that need additional support to achieve.

WHEN CONFIRMATION OF ACHIEVEMENT CANNOT BE MADE

There will be occasions where it is not possible to confirm that a student has met the required level of proficiency to pass their placement overall. This can be for a number of reasons.

The Student Has 'Not Achieved' one or More Assessment Elements

In this situation there are one or more elements within the PAD that the student has been assessed on where they have been 'graded' as 'not achieved'. If any of these elements were assessed by the practice assessor then they will have the evidence of why the student was unsuccessful and should have recorded that in the PAD. If the assessment was made by a practice supervisor a discussion should have taken place with the practice assessor so that they can be assured that the assessment was fair and reliable and appropriate evidence is provided to support the decision. The practice assessor will be required to identify in their final interview which of the specific assessment elements the student did not achieve, state why the student was 'graded' as 'not achieved' and what help and support the student will need on their next placement to enable them to be successful at the next attempt.

If there had been an indication that the student would not achieve the assessment element during the placement then an action plan should also have been written which is additional evidence to support the decision made. Chapter 8 discussed the process that should be followed when a student is not meeting the progress expected and how to develop action plans. However, there may be occasions where a student had been making the expected progress but then failed to achieve the element just before the end of the placement and there has been insufficient time to agree an action plan. For example, the student does something completely unexpected such as inappropriate conduct with a patient/service user or member of staff or decides to administer drugs without supervision. In these situations the relevant professional value may be used to record 'not achieved' against or if a previous proficiency was passed this could be updated to a 'not achieved'.

Another reason for students not having achieved all the required assessment elements is not because they were assessed and 'graded' as 'not achieved' but because it was not possible to provide the learning opportunities for the student to be assessed on a specific proficiency or proficiencies.

No Opportunity to Be Assessed on One or More Elements

Whilst the NMC proficiencies are generic and expected to be achieved by all fields it is possible that some may be more difficult to achieve in certain types of placements. If it has not been possible to identify an alternative way for the student to achieve one of the assessment elements (via an outreach placement or through simulation) this should be noted in the student's PAD as part of the documentation of the final feedback as an action for the next placement.

WHEN THE STUDENT HAS FAILED TO ACHIEVE

In the last chapter we looked at 'failure to fail' and discussed the issues associated with practice assessors making poor and inaccurate assessment decisions, often based on poor evidence or not understanding what was required. We discussed the fact that 'failure to fail' is also often the result of practice assessors failing to identify and assist underperforming students early in the placement and then providing support to the student through agreed action plans for the remaining time on the placement. It is at the final interview that 'failure to fail' takes place. Without evidence to support the final assessment decision to say that the student has not met the requirements for a pass, practice assessors may be tempted to pass students who have not reached a satisfactory standard.

An Incomplete Assessment

We have already discussed the need to ensure that by the time of the final interview the assessment decisions for the majority if not all of the assessment elements that needed to be assessed should have already been reached. Unfortunately, some practice assessors will reach the final interview without having completed a continuous assessment of all the different elements the student needs to be assessed on. This creates a situation which can be problematic. Where a practice assessor reaches the final interview without a clear picture of what the decision will be regarding the assessment judgement then the fairness and accuracy of the assessment is questionable.

Typically this situation may arise when a practice assessor reaches the final interview and realises that one or more elements within the PAD have not been assessed throughout the placement. This is usually down to not following the steps of the assessment process throughout the placement.

This can be avoided by conducting a thorough initial interview where all assessment requirements are discussed and plans put in place to undertake appropriate learning experiences. In Chapter 5 we discussed a 'checklist' for the initial interview that can help ensure all elements that need to be assessed are identified. In Chapter 7 we identified that at the midpoint interview there should have been a thorough review of progress on all elements. If progress is not being made or evidence of progress is not available, then this should be picked up and planned for in the second half of the placement. Where these two formal stages of the interview process are completed then there is far less chance of important elements being missed.

If this does happen then it is an indication that the assessment process may not have been followed. Whatever the reason may be, a failure to ensure that the student was on track to complete all the required elements creates enormous pressure on a practice assessor as the student will be expecting that an assessment decision is going to be made. Under such circumstances a practice assessor may panic, they recognise that a decision needs to be made but have little or no evidence of the student's proficiency. At this point the practice assessor has to make a decision on what action they will take. Possible decisions and their consequences are described below.

Decision One

The practice assessor could administer a last-minute, sudden test of the student's knowledge. They may ask one or a series of questions designed to 'test' knowledge. The student's answers under these circumstances will form the basis of their assessment decision.

Consequence of Decision One

Basing an assessment decision on a last-minute, one-off test proves nothing at all. If the student manages to produce the correct answer this only provides evidence that on one occasion the student has given a correct response. It provides no evidence whatsoever that future actions or responses will also be correct. There is little reliability or validity in this judgement. Alternatively, if the student responds with an incorrect answer this is not evidence in itself that the student will be incorrect every time as nerves will come into play when it is a last-minute surprise assessment. So whilst a one-off assessment provides limited evidence of a student's knowledge, skill and attitudes in relation to an area of practice, practice assessors who have not undertaken continuous assessment throughout the placement may be tempted to rely on a questionable approach to assessment to determine an assessment result. Clearly, if continuous assessment has not been undertaken this approach provides a very poor option and is not complaint with the NMC requirements that assessment is a continuous process based on feedback from a range of sources.

Decision Two

The practice supervisor could choose to pass the student on the outstanding elements with no specific evidence of their achievement. A practice assessor who is under pressure to reach a decision with no evidence on which to base that decision may be tempted to pass the student anyway on the basis that they have not heard anything to say the student is not proficient. At the time it may seem like the best option, and while it may not be accurate, valid or reliable, it is also unlikely to cause any conflict. A practice assessor may be tempted to justify this course of action based on a belief that if the decision is incorrect then 'someone else' will pick it up with the student at a later stage, especially if a first-year student.

Consequence of Decision Two

Passing a student as achieving all the required assessment elements without evidence, either out of guilt or wishing to avoid conflict is a serious failure of a practice assessor's professional accountability and responsibility. Hoping that 'someone else' will review the assessment at a later date creates serious problems for any future practice supervisors and assessors, and denies the student the help and support they require. If the non-evidence-based pass occurs on the student's final placement, this decision then becomes confirmation that the student can progress to registration.

Decision Three

The practice assessor could choose to do no assessment at all. When a practice assessor realises they have not assessed a learning outcome they may feel that the only option open to them is to avoid the assessment altogether. In other words, if they haven't got the evidence to support an assessment decision they may choose to just not complete the assessment paperwork. Such a situation will no doubt cause conflict as the student will be expecting an assessment decision. Unless they have been informed otherwise, they will be expecting to pass their elements they have been assessed upon. They will not be expecting to hear that their practice assessor missed something in the PAD and is therefore unwilling to make a decision at all.

Consequence of Decision Three

While it might be very tempting to do nothing if something has been missed this can cause serious repercussions. The whole point of the student undertaking a practice placement is so that they may be provided with the types of learning experiences that allow for assessment of their proficiency. If a student reaches the end of a placement and their performance has not been assessed this does raise the question as to what has happened during the placement. The likely outcome is that the student will be deferred by the university and be given a further opportunity to be assessed on the outstanding elements either by returning to this placement or undertaking it on another placement. If this is their final placement then this will delay the completion of the student's programme.

Decision Four

The practice supervisor could choose to fail the student based on the fact that there is no evidence of achievement, particularly in assessment documents where the only option is to record if the student has 'achieved' or 'not achieved' the required assessment element. This approach could be appealing as a course of action. In this circumstance the practice assessor may decide that if they cannot confirm the student has 'achieved' then the only alternative is 'not achieved'.

Consequence of Decision Four

While there may be a view that this is the most 'technically' correct option based on the circumstances, very few practice assessors would be willing to fail a student based on a failure to assess all the required elements. This action is likely to cause conflict and a student could appeal the decision at the university as due process has not been followed as they have not been given an opportunity to demonstrate proficiency in the required elements. In this situation a discussion with the academic assessor is needed. If a student has passed everything, they have been assessed on but the opportunity to be assessed on an assessment element was not available or it was missed then this can become an action for the next placement. The student has still passed overall as they have met the criteria for the elements they have been assessed upon.

While it is quite clear that none of these options are attractive, it is also hopefully clear that the last option is the most appropriate. Quite clearly a practice assessor cannot justify passing a student based on poor evidence, or passing a student based on no evidence. Decisions one and two are therefore not congruent with their professional accountability. Nor is decision three as the student has not failed to achieve any of the elements they have been assessed on they just have not been assessed on elements needed to make it a complete assessment. This leaves decision four as the most appropriate response. Contacting the university will not only provide support for the practice assessor but also ensure that the student is supported through this time.

THE STUDENT'S RESPONSIBILITY IN THE ASSESSMENT PROCESS

Each student also has a responsibility in monitoring their own progress and ensuring that all assessment elements are being assessed. Where it has been identified that not all the assessment requirements are achievable they should proactively seek university guidance with their practice supervisor or assessor if it cannot be realised. They should also be monitoring their progress in achieving the required elements within the PAD and alert their practice supervisor or assessor if nothing is being signed off during the placement. e-PADs will have dashboards or alert systems that identify timescales for completion if required elements are missed which is very helpful for busy staff. Some students may lack confidence to raise concerns that not everything will be completed on time not wishing to bother their staff. However, most practice supervisors and assessors will have met students who will constantly chase them to complete their PAD. Regular meetings with the student to review the progress in completing the different elements in the PAD can reassure them and also ensures nothing is missed. This ensures that the final assessment can proceed without any problems and all the required documentation can be completed.

ENDING ON A HIGH NOTE

The final interview is the ideal opportunity to encourage the student to continue to develop both personally and professionally. Through reflection on the placement the practice assessor has an opportunity of hearing from the student about the events and circumstances they have valued the most during the course of their placement. Perhaps they were encouraged by something that the practice supervisor or assessor said or did that has made a positive lasting impression. It is important to recognise this feedback and be proud of these achievements. The influence a practice supervisor and a practice assessor can have on a student's future performance and motivation to improve cannot be underestimated.

HANDING OVER TO NEXT PRACTICE ASSESSOR

The process for handing over to the next practice assessor will have been agreed by practice partners and the university. At a minimum the practice assessor must ensure that:

- All sections in the PAD and OAR have been completed including signatures or confirming your name and email address if an e-PAD.
- All actions in an action plan have been completed and there is commentary on the outcomes, with identification of any further development needs the student may have if needed.
- The student's strengths and areas for further development are clearly recorded.

Depending on whether it is known where the student will be placed next time a more personal hand over may be possible with the next practice assessor.

Reflection on Your Experience

While the final interview might signal the end of the placement for the student, for the practice assessor it is often just a brief pause before the next student. However, it is an opportunity for a practice assessor to self-evaluate their own performance. Chapter 13 provides some ideas for evaluating your own performance.

When supporting a student in practice, there are effectively two people being assessed. While it is true that you are assessing the student; your own ability, skill and professionalism as a practice supervisor or assessor is also under scrutiny by the student. Each time you support a student on their placement you have a valuable opportunity to reflect on your own performance. This is an important part of your own professional development and can give you more confidence and enhance your own supervision and assessment skills.

Action Points

1. Ensure you are familiar with the practice assessment document (or how to use the e-PAD) and ongoing achievement record before a student arrives. If there are any queries, ask for guidance from the university.
2. Plan for the final interview and assessment by blocking out time in the day or recording the event in the off-duty.
3. Inform the academic assessor of the proposed date and time for the final interview so they can arrange to attend.
4. If a placement does not go well with a student ask the Link Lecturer if you can discuss the events that took place and what actions can be taken to ensure better experiences for future students.
5. Read the supporting information on standards for student supervision and assessment on the NMC website: https://www.nmc.org.uk/supporting-information-on-standards-for-student-supervision-and-assessment/

Chapter 10

Supporting Students With Additional Needs

Chapter Outline

INTRODUCTION

The purpose of this chapter is to explore the support offered to students with additional needs. Unsurprisingly, nursing attracts a wide range of people,

A Nurse's Survival Guide to Supervising and Assessing. https://doi.org/10.1016/B978-0-7020-8147-7.00010-7

many of whom may have additional needs, and it is not unusual that many have also been the recipients of nursing care, which led them to choose nursing as a career. Universities are seeing increasing numbers of students who have declared one or more disabilities on their university application form. In 2018–19, 15.9% of students who enrolled on nursing courses at university had declared a disability (HESA, 2019). Students with a specific learning difference (SpLD) make up the majority of students declaring a disability, with mental health difficulties being the second most common disability declared by students, with the numbers increasing each year. Under the Equality Act 2010 students who have declared a disability may require reasonable adjustments both at university and in practice to remove barriers to their learning or additional support to ensure that they are not disadvantaged. In addition, there are a number of students who have additional needs who either do not have physical or mental health impairments or do not see themselves as disabled but may have additional needs that require reasonable adjustments. A disability is a protected characteristic under the Equality Act 2010. There are also other protected characteristics under the Equality Act, such as pregnancy and religion, that may also require reasonable adjustments or accommodations to be made.

This chapter will look at what the Equality Act 2010 means for staff in placements that support students. The types of additional needs that students may have when in practice will be identified and the impact that they may have on learning in practice settings discussed. Some of the more common reasonable adjustments that can be implemented for a student in practice will also be identified. The aim is to identify the skills that practice supervisors and assessors require when responding to a student who discloses that they require reasonable adjustments, including the skills to assess and support students in a way that is fair and transparent.

DEFINITIONS AND TERMINOLOGY

It is essential to consider very careful the terminology used in relation to people with additional needs, as the majority of people who declare a disability do not see themselves as disabled. A *disability* is when a person has a physical or mental impairment that has a 'substantial' and 'long-term' negative effect on their ability to undertake normal daily activities (Equality Act 2010).

Models of Disability

Different models of disability offer different ways of looking at disability, and therefore influence how a person might respond to a disabled person. The first two models below are the ones most commonly used: the medical model and the social model. The World Health Organization (WHO) offers a third view, a framework that aims to blend these two models.

The Medical Model of Disability

The medical model sees a disability as the individual's problem, with the person dependent on others and needing to be either cured or cared for. In this model the focus is on the negatives: what the disabled person cannot do (walk, read text, hear, etc.).

The Social Model

The social model was developed by disabled people in response to the medical model, which is seen as segregating disabled people from the rest of society. With the social model, disability is not an individual's problem; rather, it is a social issue, with the environment disabling the individual. Barriers that can prevent disabled people from participating in society include:

- attitudinal barriers
- physical barriers
- policies or procedural barriers
- communication barriers.

For example, on a busy ward, a telephone has not been designed to be adjustable for a person with a hearing impairment and so will prevent that person from answering the phone.

The International Classification of Functioning, Disability and Health (WHO, 2002)

The International Classification of Functioning, Disability and Health (ICF) focuses on the level of a person's health and how that impacts on their ability to function in society, as opposed to focussing on a disability, which places people in a separate category from those who are healthy. In the framework, a health disorder or disease (which includes both physical and psychological conditions) may impact on an individual's body functions or structure, which in turn may impact on their ability to undertake certain activities. A health disorder may also impact on a person's ability to participate in life situations. In addition, there are contextual factors that can impact on an individual's ability to participate in life situations. These may be environmental factors (such as how buildings are designed, social attitudes, and legal and social structures) or personal factors in the way the individual responds to and manages their disability (age, gender, coping styles, social background, and so on). Disability therefore involves dysfunctioning in one or more areas related to impairments, activity limitations and participation restrictions (WHO, 2002).

Disabled Person or Person With a Disability

How we refer to people has a significant impact on their well-being and feeling of inclusion. A person with an impairment may not see themselves as disabled. There are differing views on the correct terms to be used and people have individual preferences. For example, some organisations will use the term *disabled people*, while others will use *persons with disabilities*. The first recognises that the person has been dis-abled from effective participation in society due to the societal barriers that exist. Terms that should never be used are

- suffering from,
- victim of,
- medical labels such as *dyslexic student* or *epileptic student*; rather say, a student with dyslexia or epilepsy.

Whilst it is essential to be sensitive to how discussions with a student who has disclosed a disability are managed, the safety of patients and service users are always the first priority.

WHAT IS MEANT BY AN ADDITIONAL NEED?

Using the WHO framework above, a person with an additional need is a person who may require reasonable adjustments to be made due to:

- Activity Limitations – difficulty in executing certain activities.
- Participation Restrictions – a problem or problems an individual may experience in involvement in life situations.
- Environmental Factors – changes in the physical, social and/or attitudinal environment in which the individual lives and conducts their life. This includes at university and on placements.

Attitudes to disabled students will be influenced by culture, background, education, and ethnicity. Nurses care for people with physical, psychological and sensory impairments. It is therefore easy to fall into the trap of seeing a disabled student as a person needing to be cared for (the medical model) and requiring them to 'fit in' within the existing structures and processes. The social model approach is very different, as the focus is on removing the barriers that prevent the student from participating fully in their placement. The social model is linked to ideas of inclusivity and widening participation, looking at ways to overcome challenges and move forward. The WHO framework acknowledges the best of both models, as there will be situations where elements of the medical model may be appropriate due to the way that the student's health condition impacts on their ability to function and may require medically based interventions.

All public organisations have a legal duty to promote equality and address inequalities under the Equality Act 2010 and therefore practice supervisors and assessors require an understanding of what this means for the way they support students in practice.

THE EQUALITY ACT 2010

The Equality Act 2010 applies to England, Scotland and Wales only. In Northern Ireland there are a number of different equality laws applying to different characteristics, including the Disability Discrimination Act, 1995, which can be found on the website for the Equality Commission for Northern Ireland. England, Scotland and Wales have different organisations that provide help and support related to the Equality Act, which can be found on the internet.

The Equality Act 2010 provides protection against discrimination. Discrimination can be direct or indirect, but in essence it relates to a person being treated less favourably because of that person's protected characteristic. The duty applies to a number of different organisations, including health and care providers such as hospitals and care homes and schools, colleges and other education providers. Public bodies have due regard to the need to:

- eliminate discrimination
- advance equality of opportunity
- foster good relations between different people when carrying out their activities.

The Act identifies nine protected characteristics:

- age
- disability
- gender reassignment
- marriage or civil partnership (in employment only)
- pregnancy and maternity
- race
- religion or belief
- sex
- sexual orientation.

Any discrimination that takes place in relation to any of the above characteristics is unlawful and includes:

- direct discrimination
- discrimination arising from disability
- victimisation
- harassment.

Direct Discrimination

This means treating a person less favourably than another person who is not disabled, solely on the grounds of their disability. This often occurs due to stereotypical assumptions or prejudice; for example, turning down an applicant to a nursing course because they have a disability even though they have met all the admission criteria. Equally, if a hospital refused to allow students with a hearing impairment or dyslexia to have placements with them then that would also be direct discrimination.

Disability-related Discrimination

In this case discrimination occurs for a disability-related reason, whereby the disabled person is treated less favourably for a reason related to their disability rather than the disability itself and it is not possible to show that that reason is justified. For example, failing a student in their practice assessment because they write slowly due to their disability would be disability-related discrimination, as there is no requirement within the standards of proficiency for students to be able to complete patient/client documentation within a specified timeframe.

Victimisation

Victimisation is unlawful and relates to someone being victimised if they make or support an allegation of disability discrimination, regardless of whether that person is themselves disabled or not.

Harassment

The harassment provision protects the disabled person from behaviour that creates an environment that the person perceives as hostile, intimidating, degrading, humiliating or offensive. This could be, for example, making jokes or derogatory remarks about their disability, blocking wheelchair access, or interfering with any special support equipment they use.

REASONABLE ADJUSTMENTS

The Equality Act 2010 requires changes or adjustments to be made to enable disabled persons to access education, employment, housing, and goods and services (shops, banks, leisure centres, etc.). There is no definitive list of what constitutes a reasonable adjustment, as this will depend on the disability, how the individual manages it, and the nature of the work activities the disabled person is involved in. Examples particularly relevant to students are:

- making adjustments to premises
- altering a student's hours in placement
- assigning a student to an appropriate placement that can meet their needs
- allowing the student to take time off during placement for rehabilitation, assessment or treatment
- giving, or arranging for, training or mentoring (whether for the disabled person or any other person)
- acquiring or modifying equipment
- modifying instructions or reference manuals
- modifying procedures for testing or assessment
- providing a reader, British sign language (BSL) signer or interpreter
- providing supervision or other support.

However, consideration will need to be given to the practicality of the adjustments, the health and safety implications for the student and others, as well as the financial or other resources of the organisation. For a placement, the practice supervisor and practice assessor may be involved in identifying potential barriers to the student's learning and the possible reasonable adjustments to overcome or remove any of these barriers for the student. They will be required to implement the adjustments that have been agreed as reasonable for the student.

It is important to note that the university and placement providers also have an *anticipatory duty*. This means that the university and placement providers should have in place systems and processes for making reasonable adjustments in anticipation of having disabled students, and that they do not wait until a disabled student arrives. For example, universities will have in place a policy on assessment processes that will include provisions for adjustments to examination processes. Students who have dyslexia, for instance, may require extra time to complete an examination and should not have assessment submission dates too close together.

Adjustments/processes or equipment that are likely be in place in most healthcare organisations are:

- access ramps
- accessible toilets
- parking bays for disabled people
- loop systems for hearing aid users
- information booklets in large font or different-coloured paper
- taped handovers for people with visual impairments
- flashing phones/alarms for people with hearing impairments
- text phones
- computers.

We will come back to reasonable adjustments later in the chapter.

DISABILITY AND THE NURSING AND MIDWIFERY COUNCIL

The NMC's prime function is to safeguard the public. It does this by setting the standards for education programmes, monitoring the quality of those programmes and giving guidance and advice to the professions. The NMC do not bar anyone with disability/ies from entering nursing and midwifery programmes. They do set requirements to *ensure that a student's health is sufficient to enable safe and effective practice* (NMC, 2018c, p. 8). To ensure this all students are required to be cleared for practice by the occupational health department, who will also identify if any reasonable adjustments are required. The NMC also requires both the education institution and their placement providers to ensure that they themselves meet the requirements of the Equality Act.

Disability legislation requires that the way a course is designed must aim to ensure it is accessible to students with disabilities and must anticipate and remove potential barriers. The university therefore has to be compliant with this legislation for all the courses that they run.

The NMC identify a number of responsibilities that the university and placement providers have for students in relation to both equality and diversity. They must ensure that all students:

3.11 have their diverse needs respected and taken into account across all learning environments, with support and adjustments provided in accordance with equalities and human rights legislation and good practice

3.12 are protected from discrimination, harassment and other behaviour that undermines their performance or confidence

3.13 are provided with information and support which encourages them to take responsibility for their own mental and physical health and wellbeing

3.14 are provided with the learning and pastoral support necessary to empower them to prepare for independent, reflective professional practice (NMC, 2018e, p. 9)

In addition, for practice placements both the university and practice partners must take account of students' individual needs and personal circumstances when allocating their practice learning including making reasonable adjustments for students with disabilities (NMC, 2018c, p. 10).

All students are required to declare both good health and good character when they apply for a nursing course and again at the start of each year of their course, and when applying to join the NMC register. The NMC is very clear that neither a health condition and/or a disability would necessarily prevent someone from becoming a nurse.

Each applicant to a university who declares a disability is considered on an individual basis to identify what, if any, reasonable adjustments would be required to remove any barriers to them undertaking the programme and achieving the competence standards required. The focus is always on whether or not a student will be able to practice safely and effectively. The standards of proficiency therefore require that at the point of registration, *registered nurses, midwives and nursing associates must understand the professional responsibility to adopt a healthy lifestyle to maintain the level of fitness and wellbeing required to meet people's needs for mental and physical care* (NMC, 2019b). Students therefore also have a responsibility to maintain their own health, and this would include adhering to any guidance provided to maintain their health status.

THE IMPLICATIONS OF THE EQUALITY ACT FOR SUPPORTING STUDENTS IN PRACTICE

Put simply, the placement provider and the staff who support students in practice are legally required to comply with the Equality Act 2010, and professionally required to comply with the standards set by the NMC, which includes ensuring experiences are inclusive and that they support the diverse needs for each student. As part of this the placement provider will provide equality and diversity training that will encompass information on disabilities which all staff are required to complete.

The responsibilities of practice supervisors and practice assessors therefore are to:

- complete statutory/mandatory training on equality and diversity and complete updates as required
- identify any gaps in their knowledge regarding their role in working with and supporting both students and colleagues who have a disability and seek to rectify those gaps
- seek guidance and support from the university or senior colleagues at work when unsure how to proceed if supporting a student who has declared a disability
- support students with a disability, treating them no less favourably than they would any other student
- implement reasonable adjustments to ensure that students are not discriminated against.

DISCLOSURE

It is quite possible to be supporting a student and be unaware that they have a disability. This may be because it is a hidden impairment or disability and they have decided not to disclose it. Often this is because a student feels able to manage their disability without any adjustments being required and so did not see the need to inform anyone. However, there are students who do not tell their staff in practice about their disability because their previous experiences of disclosing have resulted in less than positive attitudes from others, either towards their disability or to disabled students in general.

Informing another person about a disability is called *disclosure*. Students have the right not to disclose their disability or to decide whom they wish to disclose to. If they restrict who is informed, they are advised that this may limit the support that the university or practice can provide.

The university and placement providers, as public bodies, are required to provide opportunities for students to disclose throughout their programme. This is not a one-off event and it is important that information for disabled students is widely available so that they are aware of their rights and the processes available to them to access support. At the very least, information will be provided in programme/course handbooks and on the university website. The orientation checklist in a student's practice assessment document (PAD) also includes an opportunity for a student to disclose their disability, or other reasons for reasonable adjustments.

What Happens Following Disclosure?

Students may disclose their disability on their application form, at interview, or at any point during the programme. However, many students are not identified as having dyslexia until after they start their nursing programme. This usually occurs after a member of academic staff has identified that they may be dyslexic after seeing their academic writing or the student has undertaken a test for dyslexia.

When disclosed on the application form the university will usually contact the student and invite them to meet with a Disability Team Advisor to discuss the support that they will need at their interview and whilst studying at the university. In the case of nursing students, they will also need to discuss the support that the student will require during their practice placements. If a student discloses after starting the programme, they will be referred to the Disability Team at that point. For students who have disclosed a mental health condition, referral will include referral to a Mental Health Advisor.

When the Disability Team Advisor meets with the student, they will discuss with the student who at the university and elsewhere will need to be informed about their disability/ies in order for reasonable adjustments to be put in place. The student will be asked to sign consent as to whom disclosure can be shared with, and if they limit who can be told they will be informed that this will affect the level of support that can be provided. In some cases, the student may be happy to share details regarding the reasonable adjustments they require, but not details of their impairment or disability.

The Disability Team Adviser will also be able to advise the student on the disability support funding that may be available to them and how to apply for it. This money is to cover additional costs that may arise because of the student's disability and is not means-tested. The type of funding allowances available are:

- specialist equipment allowance, for example computer, specialist furniture, electronic stethoscopes
- non-medical helper's allowance – to pay for a support worker, communication support worker or personal assistant
- general expenditure allowance
- travel allowance – to pay for travel expenses that are additional to those other students pay for (e.g. taxi fare rather than bus fare).

The student and the Disability Team Advisor will then draw up an agreement of the reasonable adjustments required; this may be called an Individual Support Plan or Statement of Support Needs and will address adjustments the student requires at the university and in practice placements.

It is the responsibility of the student to disclose if they require any reasonable adjustments when they attend practice. If a student requires significant adjustments, then the university, with the permission of the student, will work with the student and the placement to discuss the adjustments needed. For significant adjustments this may include a meeting with the Disability Team Advisor and/ or a specialist advisor such as an Advisory Teacher for Deaf Students to discuss the reasonable adjustments that the student will require whilst on practice placements. It may also be necessary to identify whether there are any difficulties with certain types of placements due to the nature of care delivery or where they are geographically located. Ideally, the placement pathway for the whole programme will be looked at in advance; to identify any specific placements that may pose significant challenges so there is forward planning to prepare the adjustments needed for them.

General factors to consider when considering each placement might be:

- distance from transport links
- accessibility at the actual placement
- noise levels
- light levels
- flexibility of work patterns
- the placement speciality.

It is important to remember that the focus on making reasonable adjustments is on what needs to be put in place to enable the student to meet the competence standards of the programme. Competence standards themselves will not be changed, but how the student is expected to perform and be assessed against these may need to be adjusted. For example:

- A student with a hearing impairment is required to demonstrate competence in taking baseline observations. She achieves this on a ward placement by using an electronic monitor with a visual display to show blood pressure. There is no requirement in the competence standards that she has to specifically use a standard stethoscope.
- A student with dyscalculia is allowed to use a calculator when calculating drug dosages.
- A student who has been diagnosed with dyslexia has extra time in the working day to undertake and complete a patient or service user's nursing care notes. There is no requirement in the competence standards that he has to complete them within a specified time frame.

The Responsibility of the Practice Supervisor and Assessor in Relation to Disclosure

Practice supervisors and practice assessors have a responsibility to create an environment in which all students feel comfortable to discuss confidential information with them. This includes enabling them to feel comfortable disclosing their disability and/or discussing the reasonable adjustments that they may require. At the initial interview it is essential to ask the student whether there are any reasonable adjustments that they require whilst on placement. This gives them the opportunity to disclose a disability and discuss reasonable adjustments required. In some cases, a student may prefer to discuss reasonable adjustments without disclosing their actual disability. This is their right. They should share their individual learning plan or statement of support needs so that the adjustments required can be identified and implemented.

Since a student can disclose at any time in their programme, there are a number of possible scenarios for when a student may be identified as requiring reasonable adjustments:

1. The student has disclosed at the university and reasonable adjustments have been agreed upon and the student:
   a. Arranges to meet with their practice supervisor or assessor in advance or on the first day of their placement to discuss the reasonable adjustments they require.
   b. Decides not to inform anyone until later in the placement when they feel comfortable with their practice supervisor or assessor or they wait until they run into difficulties related to their disability.
2. The student has not disclosed to the university – no reasonable adjustments are agreed and the student:
   a. Discloses that they have a disability during their placement.
   b. Does not disclose that they have a disability, but it is believed by staff members supporting them that they may have.

Let's look at each of these scenarios in turn.

1a. The student discloses at the university and reasonable adjustments have been agreed in advance.
   The ideal situation is that the student will have visited their placement prior to it starting so that the adjustments required can be discussed in advance. Depending on what adjustments are required and who the student has agreed this can be shared with, people who may be involved at the first meeting could be:
   ● The student
   ● The practice supervisor and/or assessor and/or manager of the placement
   ● The student's personal tutor/the Link Lecturer
   ● The Disability Team Advisor from the university
   ● The person with responsibility for equality and diversity in your organisation.
1b. The student discloses at the university and reasonable adjustments have been agreed in advance, but they do not inform anyone until later in the placement.
   As soon as a student discloses that they require reasonable adjustments then the reasonable adjustments agreed have to be put in place. Support may be requested from the Link Lecturer or personal tutor to ensure appropriate adjustments are implemented.

2a. The student discloses a disability on placement but doesn't have any reasonable adjustments agreed with the university.

Sometimes the student has chosen not to disclose to the university either because they believe they can manage any adjustments required without additional help or did not appreciate that they might require reasonable adjustments to be made when on placement until they got there. For example, a student who has diabetes may need regular meal breaks. Having regular meal breaks is a reasonable adjustment; however, there are additional questions to consider. For example:

- What happens if your diabetes becomes unstable?
- What are the signs we should be aware of?
- What actions should we take?
- If you should have a hypoglycaemic attack or become unwell is there anyone we should contact?
- Who else on this placement can I tell that you have diabetes?

If the student requests that no one else is to be informed about their diabetes, then it will be important to discuss what information can be shared – for example, informing staff that the student requires regular meal breaks without giving the reason why. However, in restricting the information that can be shared should the student have a hypoglycaemic episode, this could have serious implications for them if other staff do not know and so may not recognise what is happening. The student may therefore decide that they will inform people on a need-to-know basis.

2b. A student may decide not to disclose their disability but it is either apparent because it can be seen (e.g. the student wears a hearing aid) or it may be that it is believed that they may have a hidden disability which has become apparent from their performance on the placement (e.g. dyslexia).

By asking all students whether they require any reasonable adjustments at the start of their placement this can be pre-empted. If they have a disability that is obvious, then under the Equality Act 2010 reasonable adjustments must be put in place; however, this could be difficult unless it is clear exactly what adjustments the student requires and may require a discussion with the student and the university and a referral to the university disability team.

If it is believed that a student may have a hidden disability based upon their performance or behaviour on the placement, but they have not disclosed a disability nor requested reasonable adjustments, this will require sensitive handling. Where there are concerns regarding any student's performance, discussing the concerns with them and asking if there are any factors that may be affecting the student that could as a consequence be impacting on their performance is important. It is important to document any discussions with the student in their practice assessment document and agree on clear action plans. If there are significant concerns regarding performance or a disability is then identified, then contact the Link Lecturer or Academic Assessor and invite them to the meeting with the student.

> ! At the initial interview always ask students whether there are any reasonable adjustments they may require during their placement.

While on their placement it is quite possible that students may learn more about their disability/ies through being involved in caring for people with the same or similar disabilities. This could be viewed positively by the student or may create anxiety about their own disability. It is important to be sensitive to this and offer students the opportunity to discuss this experience with them.

Some students may need to attend support sessions during their placement: study skills for dyslexia, counselling or mentoring. It is important that they are allowed to attend these as these will be part of the reasonable adjustments identified for them. It will be necessary to discuss with the Link Lecturer whether this time counts as part of their clinical hours or whether an agreement has been made to enable the student to make up any missed time to attend these meetings.

Disclosure and Confidentiality

If a student discloses a disability to you, there are a number of issues to consider around confidentiality. Details about a person's disability cannot be shared with anyone else without their consent. It is therefore important to discuss with the student whom they have already disclosed this to and who this can be shared with on placement.

If this is the first time they have disclosed to anyone and they request that no one else is informed it is important to explain that whilst it is possible to make reasonable adjustments in the way that the student is supported, any adjustments that require specialist equipment or require actions by the placement provider or by the university may not be possible to put in place immediately. Explain that by informing the disability support team at the university a more co-ordinated approach can be taken and will also allow the student to access specific funds through the disability student allowance, if needed, which can help provide specialist equipment, funding for a personal assistant or travel expenses.

If the student has an individual support plan in place but does not wish anyone else to know about their disability, then a discussion is needed on how they want to share this information with other colleagues that they will be working with. Again, it is important that the student understands that limiting who knows can impact on the level of support provided.

The Student's Responsibility in Placement

The Equality Act 2010 clearly sets out the rights of people with disabilities. However, with rights come responsibilities and there are certain responsibilities that the student has in relation to their disability, which include:

- To accept that if they do not disclose their disability to key staff then this will limit the support that can be provided.
- To be actively involved in identifying the reasonable adjustments they require and the development of their individual support plan.
- To inform relevant staff where there are problems with implementing the agreed adjustments, or if they are insufficient, to enable them to participate fully in the learning experiences.
- To access the Disability Team at the university and any other support networks that are available.

In most cases the student will be an expert on their disability and how it affects them and so it is imperative that their experience of what strategies and adjustments work for them are discussed and taken into account. No two students with the same disability will necessarily require the same adjustments.

REASONABLE ADJUSTMENTS FOR SPECIFIC IMPAIRMENTS OR DISABILITIES

This section looks briefly at the more common disabilities/impairments that students may require reasonable adjustments for in practice.

Chronic Fatigue Syndrome

Students may have difficulties with concentration, handling a lot of tasks at once, stamina or memory. Examples of reasonable adjustments which students may find helpful include:

- adjustment to shift times and patterns
- regular breaks
- being allocated a smaller group of patients/clients to care for
- placements which do not require long travelling times
- use of notes/checklists.

Diabetes Mellitus

Students are encouraged to inform the staff in practice about their condition, particularly where it may not be well controlled, and explain how they might behave before they have a hypoglycaemic episode and contact details for someone if they become suddenly ill.

Examples of reasonable adjustments which students may find helpful include:

- regular meal breaks
- time off to attend hospital/doctor appointments.

Epilepsy

With epilepsy there may be unexpected relapses in the control of the condition, possibly due to the effects of longer days and the general stresses of coping with learning new skills and responsibilities in clinical areas. It is important to be aware of triggers previously not encountered. For example, where photosensitivity is a problem, photographic angiography or radiographic departments may cause difficulties. Some students may experience concentration difficulties, side effects of medication or fatigue due to lack of sleep. It is important to agree with the student what action should be taken if they experience an aura, the actions that should be taken if they experience a seizure, and how much recovery time they might need.

Reasonable adjustments are likely to focus around the avoidance of triggers. If the student knows the potential triggers for their seizures, they will need to discuss these so that help can be provided to identify/avoid the relevant departments or equipment where the triggers may be found.

Hearing Impairment

Students with a hearing impairment may experience barriers to communication in practice, such as noise levels, lighting, accents, verbal alerts and auditory alarms. It is important to discuss with the student their individual circumstances and the support they require.

Examples of reasonable adjustments which students may require are:

- equipment for taking vital signs that have visual displays, for example blood pressure and pulse monitors
- amplified stethoscopes
- vibrating alerts to signal a monitor's alarm
- vibrating alerts for fire or emergency alarms
- text telephones
- amplified telephone
- placements that are smaller/quieter without too much background noise.
- To gain experience of night duty in a placement where lights may be left on at night (e.g. A&E) or flexible shift patterns, for example undertaking twilight shifts rather than full night shifts.
- Support of a British Sign Language interpreter on placement. This would require pre-planning to identify appropriate placements and how patients or service users' consent will be managed.

Mental Health Difficulties

Mental health difficulties can fluctuate and therefore the student's support requirements may also fluctuate. At the initial interview discuss with the student what behaviour they may exhibit that would indicate that their health status is deteriorating. If a student appears to be unaware of a change in behaviour that indicates a possible relapse in their condition or exhibits mental distress which does not appear to be being managed well, this should be identified with them and appropriate coping strategies that they may have explored and how they can be implemented. Should this not be sufficient then the Link Lecturer or Academic Assessor may need to be contacted for further advice.

Examples of reasonable adjustments which students may find helpful include:

- flexible work patterns to enable optimum performance as some medications may make a student particularly drowsy in the morning and long shifts can create additional stresses
- modify workloads if required
- allow time off to attend hospital appointments/counselling.

Specific Learning Differences

SpLDs such as dyslexia, dysgraphia, dyspraxia, attention deficit (hyperactivity) disorder, or dyscalculia are recognised and covered as disabilities by disability legislation. SpLDs are the most common disability disclosed by students. Students with SpLD may have a range of support requirements outlined in their individual support plan for when they are on placement. Different aspects of placements may present different barriers to students with SpLD, in particular:

Memory difficulties, organisation and time management: organised attendance, remembering verbal instructions, accurate understanding of verbal instructions, completing documentation within a defined time frame, poor concentration span, learning terms and conditions, remembering names and job titles, managing diary appointment/shift times, sequencing tasks, multitasking.

Reading: reading quickly or in noisy environments, reading information on charts, recognising drug names/reading prescriptions.

Writing and spelling: spelling, clear and good presentation of written work, effective note taking, writing under time pressures, structuring and organising their thoughts in reports.

Motor skills: identifying left from right, sequencing activities when undertaking certain skills.

Numbers: drug calculations, recording observations on charts, adding up fluid charts.

It will be helpful to identify with the student potential aspects of their placement that may present barriers and discuss possible solutions/reasonable adjustments to remove barriers. This should be reviewed on a regular basis.

Examples of reasonable adjustments which students with an SpLD may find helpful include:

- regular opportunities to ask questions
- breaking down instructions into manageable steps

- repeating instructions/allowing student to write instructions down
- recorded handovers that they can go back to and listen to as needed
- providing examples of well-completed documentation
- ask the student to repeat back information or instructions to check understanding
- additional time to take notes/complete documentation
- lists of terms, abbreviations and common conditions.

The student may also bring the following with them and should be encouraged to use them if so:

- a calculator
- coloured overlays.

Visual Impairment

It is important that a student with a visual impairment has an orientation to the physical layout of the placement, preferably before the first day of the placement, to enable them to become familiar with the environment and identify any possible additional risks. Discuss with the student if the lighting levels are sufficient in the placement area for the student to be able to work night shifts, if appropriate. This is important as individuals with a visual impairment can suffer night blindness in low light levels.

Examples of reasonable adjustments that students may find helpful include:

- handouts or information for students such as an induction pack; this should be provided in their preferred format (larger font, different coloured paper)
- specialist equipment such as talking thermometers, blood pressure monitors, blood glucose monitors
- hand or stand magnifiers for reading documents
- computers with text-enlargement software
- braille note-takers
- laptops/access to computers to complete patient documentation
- recorded handovers.

ASSESSING DISABLED STUDENTS

This is probably the area that creates the most anxiety for the practice assessor, as many fear that failing a disabled student may be seen as discriminatory. However, as long the assessment is based on evidence, is objective and fair, and all reasonable adjustments have been implemented then the student will need to have demonstrated that they achieved the requirements of the proficiencies and met the assessment criteria.

As discussed earlier there is no requirement to lower the competence standards against which the student will be assessed, but different or modified assessment approaches may be required. For example, it may be necessary to give a student who has dyslexia longer to undertake an admission assessment and develop a plan of care. The assessment should focus on the proficiencies and professional values within the PAD.

The usual assessment process should be followed, which means:

- identifying and agreeing on the proficiencies to be assessed
- identifying the learning opportunities available to achieve the proficiencies
- agreeing how the reasonable adjustments will be implemented to support the student to achieve the proficiencies
- agreeing what the student will need to do to demonstrate achievement of the proficiencies
- agreeing on dates for reviews of progress.

Regular meetings are important to review progress against the agreed learning plan. When giving feedback, do not be afraid to give honest feedback but ensure that the feedback on their performance is against the agreed proficiencies and assessment criteria standards. If the student is not making the progress expected it is important to discuss with them why they think this may be. If the adjustments are not effective, they may need to be reviewed and alternative adjustments put in place. In this case it may be necessary to suspend the assessment process until the additional or revised adjustments have been made. Ensure all discussions with the student are recorded in their practice assessment document.

If the student is still not making the required progress despite reasonable adjustments, then an action plan will need to be developed, which was discussed in Chapter 8.

EVALUATING THE SUPPORT OF THE STUDENT WITH A DISABILITY

Once reasonable adjustments have been put in place it is important to monitor their effectiveness on a regular basis throughout the placement to ensure they are continuing to meet the student's needs. For example, a student with diabetes may find that despite regular meal breaks, working long days is impacting on their blood sugar levels and so they request to do a combination of early and late shifts in order to meet their practice hours. This would be a reasonable adjustment but may require a rethink of the off-duty to ensure that the student continues to be supported through the placement.

ADJUSTMENTS FOR STUDENTS WHO DO NOT HAVE A DISABILITY

There are students with other protected characteristics or additional needs that also need to be considered as they may also require reasonable adjustments to support them in practice or additional needs to be accommodated.

Students Who are Pregnant

Students who are pregnant will have had a risk assessment undertaken at the university and should bring this to their placement, preferably in advance of starting. Adjustments that are likely to be required are:

- regular meal breaks
- time off for antenatal care
- modified shifts if they have morning sickness or find it difficult to manage long shifts
- avoidance of certain chemicals or X-rays

Students With Child or Family Care Commitments

With increasing numbers of mature students entering nursing many students now have children and/or elderly family members. As students are supernumerary in practice there is the potential for some flexibility in the shifts they undertake. Where a student has significant problems due to childcare or care for family members that are not short term, a discussion should be held with the university to agree what accommodations can be made for the student that still enable effective supervision and a fair assessment to take place.

THE CONTRIBUTION OF DISABLED STUDENTS

Disabled students bring additional skills to practice settings that are not always acknowledged. They have a lived experience of disability and so can offer alternative views to the patient/service user experience and demonstrate a greater empathy in practice. Students with a SpLD have been identified as being insightful, intuitive, creative and lateral thinkers (Major & Tetley, 2019) and due to an understanding of the nature of their disability can have a higher level of self-awareness with regards to the potential safety issues. Living with a disability can develop resilience in students, an attribute which appears in two of the NMC proficiencies and is increasingly sought after by employers.

Action Points

- Ensure you complete statutory/mandatory training on diversity and equality training.
- Ask all students if they require reasonable adjustments at the start of their placement.
- Check what resources are available from the university for supporting students with a disability; these may be available on their website or as a handbook for practice supervisors and practice assessors.
- Evaluate the effectiveness of reasonable adjustments used and consider what guidance and tools can be developed for future students with a similar disability to support them.

Chapter 11

Managing Challenges When Supporting Students

Chapter Outline

INTRODUCTION

Supporting students in practice will usually go without any problems but sometimes difficulties can arise for a range of different reasons. These situations may impact on the planned learning experience you aim to provide for the student, or they can impact on your perception of students if they do not go well. Often the challenges can arise due to sudden changes in the workplace or may be because a student has differing expectations of what will happen when they are in practice. Difficulties can also arise where staff supporting students lack sufficient understanding of the course the student is undertaking or policies that apply to students or the NMC requirements that have to be met and which students must comply with. The purpose of this chapter is to explore some of the common challenges or difficulties that you may encounter in supporting students in practice and offer some practical approaches to address these challenges without compromising the quality and assessment of learning.

DEMOGRAPHIC DIFFERENCES IN NURSING

Nursing attracts a diverse range of people with students of all ages (from 18 to 50+). The diversity of each student group will vary across the UK depending in part on local populations but also on the field of practice. In general children's nursing tends to attract younger, predominantly female students, whereas mental health nursing will have a greater percentage of male students than any other field and usually they are representative of a more mature age group. In 2019, 22.6% of acceptances onto nursing courses were from 18-year-olds with 19% of acceptances in the 35 years and over age group; a rise of 12.9% from 2018 (UCAS, 2019); see Table 11.1. This upswing in applicants over 35 suggests that there is an increasing number of mature entrants who are seeing nursing as a future career choice. These students will bring significant life experience and a range of skills from their prior work experiences into nursing. Differences in ages between practice supervisors/ assessors and their students can bring both challenges and benefits, as people from these different generations can have quite diverse expectations of each other and very different sets of personal beliefs and values related to work. This diversity is to be valued but can also sometimes bring challenges within placements.

Generational Differences

It is not uncommon to hear nurses in practice say that students today are 'not like they were in my day'. This is true. The nursing profession encompasses individuals across four generations. Each of these generations will have been shaped by the world in which they grew up and so will have different attitudes to work and its value and importance in their life (Health Education England, 2019; Jones et al., 2015). There has been an increase in research into generational differences and whilst some caution is needed, as we are all individuals, it does provide evidence that is worth considering when working both with colleagues and students who are from a different generation than yourself. Box 11.1 provides a summary of the characteristics of these different generational groups. An understanding of what is important and valued by

TABLE 11.1 Acceptances to Nursing Courses in 2019

Age	% of Acceptances to Nursing Courses
18	22.6
19	12.0
20	6.4
21–24	16.1
25–29	14.0
30–34	9.8
35–39	7.7
40–44	5.8
45–49	3.4
50–54	1.6
55 and over	0.5

UCAS, 2019. Nursing by individual age. UCAS Undergraduate Sector-Level End of Cycle Data Resources 2019. Available at: https://www.ucas.com/

different generational groups and how they differ from your own can help you to understand why personal (rather than professional) values may differ. It is important to recognise that personal values around work and lifestyles that are different from your own are not wrong but can explain why students from a different generation to you may respond to situations differently than you would. At a simplistic level a 'Baby Boomer' is more likely to stay late to help out compared to a 'Generation Z'. 'Generation X' students may appear more 'needy', wanting supervision, support and reassurance with regular feedback. Generation Y and Z are much more technology-savvy and are comfortable with and use technology to both communicate and learn. When they email or message, they expect an immediate response. It has also been shown that 'Generation Z' see positive mental health as important and are more likely to feel the pressure of work and take time out because they feel stressed or overwhelmed (Pegasus, 2018).

! Review the Mind the Gap videos on YouTube by Health Education England which are excellent short cartoon videos which summarise each of the generational groups: https://bit.ly/MtGVideos

BOX 11.1 Characteristics of Different Generations

Name	Period born	Characteristics & age groups (in 2020)
Baby Boomers	1946–1964	Loyal, extremely hard-working and a team player. (56–74)
Generation X	1965–1980	Prefer structure and direction. Multitaskers. Work-life balance important. (40–55)
Generation Y 'Millennials'	1981–1995	Ambitious, high expectations. Supervision and support important to them and appreciate frequent feedback and guidance. Seek out environments that demonstrate team working and a sense of community. Like autonomy. Tech savvy. Work-life balance is paramount. (25–39)
Generation Z 'Digital natives'	1995–2010	Thrive on instant gratification and prefer information to be delivered in rapid, short bursts or 'sound bites' if it is to be understood. Seek flexibility and insist on a work-life balance. More likely to feel pressure and take time off work. (18–24)

Adapted from Health Education England (2019) and Jones et al. (2015).

THE COURSE–LIFE BALANCE

As discussed earlier the demographics of students entering nursing are changing with more mature students commencing their degrees. In some parts of the UK the majority of students starting pre-registration nursing courses are identified as mature entrants. As a consequence, we are seeing more students coming into nurse education after starting a family or having decided on a significant career change.

All of the above can lead to challenges as the student is faced with juggling the demands of family, friends and coursework commitments as well as attending practice and undertaking shift work. In addition, many students have jobs to help support them financially. This may result in some students requesting changes to shifts or declining to undertake specific shift patterns during their practice experience. While you may feel very tempted to allow students to request a specific rota out of kindness, this can result in the student not being on duty with you therefore limiting your opportunity to supervise and assess their performance. Lack of regular contact with a student can result in difficulties in picking up on a student who is not meeting the expected standard early enough to put in place actions to help them succeed.

As difficult as it may be, reinforcing the need for the student to undertake regular shifts with you is necessary. In addition, the NMC requires students to participate in the full range of care across 24 hours, including weekends and night duty (NMC, 2018c) and students can feel frustrated by what they may perceive as strict rules and regulations. However, this is an NMC and course requirement and students must achieve this by the end of their programme in order to qualify. It is a good idea to confirm with the university the expectations they have regarding students' shift patterns and ensure these policies are maintained in your practice area. This information may also be in their practice assessment document or in handbooks for practice supervisors and assessors. Some universities may issue a letter of negotiated shifts for students (or equivalent) that have a specific need for negotiated shifts for their placement to allow some flexibility to manage exceptional circumstances.

Consistency of how difficulties like this are managed is as important between placements as it is between practice supervisors and assessors, and this is not always easy to achieve. Attending education meetings within your wider organisation and at a more local level and discussing such issues is an ideal way to share good practice and agree approaches to enhance continuity across your organisation/department. Of course, there will be times that you exercise your professional judgement and allow the student to choose or swap shifts, but this must not be at the expense of their learning needs. Students must complete a minimum number of hours across the 24-hour period and failure to achieve this is not in keeping with course or NMC requirements or professional in behaviour. Persistent and consistent changes to off-duty or refusal to do certain shifts can be assessed against the relevant professional behaviour. Involvement of the Link Lecturer and/or Academic Assessor is advisable in situations like this to confirm the requirements and expectations.

! Use the initial interview to establish with the student any special circumstances the student may have that could prevent them undertaking their designated off-duty. Seek advice from the university if the student will be unable to commit to the planned off-duty for the placement.

Working While Learning

Financial hardship is a reality for many students. Under these circumstances it is not uncommon to discover that students are undertaking paid work as bank or agency healthcare assistants, which may lead to increased tiredness, reduced concentration and poor performance. If you suspect the student of working excessive hours on bank, agency or other paid employment but do not have the evidence you are advised to assess the student on the behaviour which is causing concern. For example, if the student is witnessed to fall asleep whilst on duty or is having difficulty with concentration or maintaining punctuality, then these are the areas to focus upon. If this happens with a student allocated to you then:

- Meet with the student to discuss the behaviour. Highlight which professional value(s) they are not currently meeting the expected standard for.
- Discuss what behaviours are expected and how their ongoing performance will be monitored.
- Record the incident in the student's practice assessment document, with clear details of future performance expected of the student.
- If there are concerns regarding their health and well-being, you may decide that the student should go home to sleep or rest and return to duty when fit to come back (this should be noted in their timesheet).

If you discover that your student was on duty the night before and they are now on placement during the day, immediate action needs to be taken to protect patients and the student. You should send the student home to sleep/rest until fit to return. Whether it is working excessive hours or working back-to-back shifts, you should inform the Link Lecturer and Academic Assessor so that a tripartite discussion can take place with the student when they next return to placement to discuss the concerns you have about their behaviour. Linking their behaviour to a professional value that they would not be meeting if they fall asleep in practice or work a night shift followed by attending practice on a day shift is important, as it is more likely to reinforce the seriousness of their actions. An example of a professional value this behaviour could potentially relate to is:

The student understands their professional responsibility in adopting and promoting a healthy lifestyle for the well-being of themselves and others.

Pan London Practice Learning Group (2019a)

A student who is failing to look after themselves or failing to recognise that they have a problem is potentially putting the people that they are caring for at risk and immediate action is required.

PROFESSIONAL CONDUCT

The professional values are an essential part of the practice assessment document which students are required to demonstrate in practice. However, this can sometimes be complicated by the differences between our personal and professional views of acceptable standards and expectations. It is important to communicate and inform students what your expectations and standards are as well as acting as a role model in the way that you demonstrate them in your everyday practice.

Explaining to students and role modelling how you would like them to behave is very important. Do not assume that the students are aware of what is or is not considered professional behaviour as a nurse, particularly with first-year students; it is the time they spend in practice which will help them to develop these professional behaviours. For example, consider a student on a community mental health placement who decides to make notes during the practice supervisor's discussion with the service user they were visiting. The student's aim is to capture the learning he was seeing, but the practice supervisor might see this as rude and unprofessional, wanting the student to observe and listen carefully to the interaction. A briefing before they went in would have helped the student to understand what was expected of him and to consider not only his own learning needs but how the service user might view his behaviour.

It can be difficult at times to articulate what we mean by 'behave professionally' as it encompasses a range of characteristics. However, most practice assessment documents contain a list of professional values and behaviours expected of a student which can make this easier to articulate, as it they can be used as the basis for a discussion with the student. Simple ones to start with when you have first-year students are:

- adherence to the dress code (uniform policy)
- punctuality
- informing you if they will be late/off sick
- demonstrating interest and motivation
- developing the ability to listen, ask questions and seek clarification if unclear on actions to be taken.

As many professional values are based on the *Code* (NMC, 2018a) it is useful to reference this to the student as they will be familiar with this from university as well as referencing their practice assessment document. If your student is behaving in a manner which is not meeting the expected professional values set out in their practice assessment document or in the *Code,* it is important to explain the reasons for your concerns and try to engage the student in considering an alternative approach that will meet the expectations of the practice assessment document and the *Code.*

The following are some strategies which you can try with your students.

- Using positive statements which incorporate an explanation can illustrate what we do and why. For example, try:
  - 'I would like you to be on time for duty so that you can participate in handover' instead of 'you keep missing handover because you're late'
  - 'Our patient survey tells us that our clients/service users/patients/family/ carers like to see staff wearing ID badges to help them in recognising different people' instead of 'Where's your ID badge?'
- Encourage reflection on behaviour and problem-solving using questions such as:
  - How have other staff approached X?
  - How do you think X might respond if you were to ….?

- Use role play to try out unfamiliar situations. This is a good way to practise how to conduct oneself professionally in a safe environment.

Focusing on the behaviours rather than the presenting attitude will mean that you can give concrete examples of what is or is not acceptable in someone aspiring to becoming a registered nurse.

SICKNESS AND ABSENTEEISM

There will be times when a student calls in sick or calls to say their child-care arrangements have failed and so they are unable to attend placement. Unfortunately, this is part of daily life and can be managed locally. The challenge and problems occur when the absenteeism (regardless of reason) is persistent and extended. Long periods of absence reduce the amount of time you can spend with the student to assess them fairly. It also means the student will have fewer opportunities to demonstrate evidence of their learning and achievement of their proficiencies.

It is important that the university placements office is informed of all absences on the day the student is absent regardless of the reason given by the student. This way a record is immediately kept but also the amount of absence can be tracked. If there has been no contact from the student to inform you of the reason for their absence, letting the placements office know means that they can attempt to make contact with the student to find out what has happened and ask them to call you. When the student returns to placement discuss why it is important to inform the placement if they will be absent and its relevance to the professional values expected of a nurse; ensure that their timesheet is updated showing the time missed. It is also important that the student is reminded that if they ring in to say that they will not be attending placement that they should take the name of the person whom they spoke to. Occasionally messages are not passed on so confirmation of whom they told can be helpful.

! Students must complete a minimum of 2300 hours in practice in order to register with the NMC. If they miss time in practice, this may delay their completion and ability to register with the NMC at the end of their programme.

If the student has been absent for extended periods or has been taking a lot of odd days off, consider the following actions:

- Review and double check the off-duty – does it clearly state the shifts the student did not attend and what type of absence it was? If there are gaps liaise with the staff who were on duty on those days to confirm attendance or absence.

- Inform the student's placement office of all absences – if you email the information you can copy in the Link Lecturer or education lead, so they are kept informed.
- Arrange to meet the student with the Link Lecturer/Academic Assessor on their return to placement to discuss their absence(s), implications for the completion of their practice assessment document and any plans to make the missed hours up if time allows.
- If due to the extensive absences there is insufficient time for you to make a fair and just assessment of the student's competence you must inform the Link Lecturer and Academic Assessor as soon as possible and document this in the student's practice assessment book.

Where there is clear, documented evidence of persistent absence, the university can use this to explore with the student their ability to meet the course requirements and identify whether there are any mitigating circumstances to explain them. If there are no mitigating circumstances, then there are a number of possible outcomes. The student may be failed on the relevant professional value regarding failure to communicate appropriately if unable to attend placement, or where there are serious concerns then the student may be referred to the university fitness-to-practice panel. Key to either scenario is the evidence in timesheets, the practice assessment document (PAD), and clear documentation of any discussions with the student regarding their attendance.

! The university must always be informed about students with poor attendance.

Significant Life Events

Other life events can impact on a student's engagement with practice, such as a bereavement, caring responsibilities not only for children but parents or older members of the family, or serious ill health of a family member. If you are informed by the student that a relative or friend has died, and they would like time off to grieve and travel to the funeral then this must be agreed with the university. In these situations, the student could need more time off than they initially requested, particularly for international students or students with family overseas. Leave from the course, including time off from placement, on compassionate grounds can only be authorised by the university. As a practice supervisor/assessor your role is to support the student to follow the correct reporting procedures, as well as offering the student support as you would for any member of staff.

There may be times when the student is facing difficult personal circumstances and does not wish to take time off from the placement or programme, believing that studying and attending placement will provide a distraction and a way to cope with the loss or difficulties they are facing. Many students will also be worried about missing hours on placement, aware that they will need to be made up at some point. If the student is struggling and this is impacting on their performance in practice it is advisable to liaise with the Link Lecturer or Academic Assessor as additional support can be put in place for the student. This may be through extra meetings arranged by the Link Lecturer or Academic Assessor with the student to ensure they feel supported, or they may require referral to support services at the university. Where the personal events in their life are significantly impacting their performance, a decision will need to be made as to whether the student should be withdrawn from placement. Making a fair and objective assessment decision in cases like this can be very difficult but students must be able to meet the standards required. The support of the Link Lecturer or Academic Assessor will be important to support both the practice assessor and the student in the process. Where it is deemed necessary, they can also support the decision to withdraw the student from the placement if their personal circumstances mean that they are not fit to be assessed.

SUPPORTING STUDENTS ON A SECOND ATTEMPT

Whilst the vast majority of students pass their practice assessments at the first attempt, a small number each year will not. It is therefore possible that you may be allocated a student who has to repeat the failed elements on their previous placement with you. This may be called a second attempt, retake, or retrieval placement.

What is a Second Attempt?

All university students are usually entitled to at least one further attempt of any assessment they have failed to pass. This may be called a second attempt or a retake. For a second attempt at practice the approach used is normally different from a second attempt at an assignment where the student has to rewrite their original assignment. A student who has failed their practice will have failed on one or more elements in their practice assessment document. They may have been failed on any or all of the following:

- one or more professional values
- one or more proficiencies
- an episode of care or in-placement assessment.

Most commonly it is the professional values that students are more likely to fail due to concerns around the student's professional conduct in practice, followed by failure at one or more proficiencies. The location, length and timing of a practice placement to undertake the second attempt are decided upon by the university and will be dependent on the needs of the individual student. The student may not undertake their second attempt in the same placement as the first attempt as usually both the practice assessor and student benefit from a fresh start.

Each university will have different regulations around assessments and as students normally have two or more placements in each academic year the student could fail in the first or second (or even third) placement. If a student fails elements in their practice assessment document (PAD) on the first placement they would need to pass (or retrieve) them on their next placement. If a student fails elements on their final placement for the year (or part of the programme), depending on university regulations they may be able to retrieve the failed elements on an additionally arranged placement before the next year/part or in the first placement in the next year/part of their programme.

The Role of the Practice Supervisor and Practice Assessor for a Second Attempt

Supporting a student who has previously failed elements in their PAD can be quite challenging. The student may enter the placement with low self-esteem or feeling very anxious and worried. Essentially, your role as a practice supervisor or assessor will not alter. You will still be expected to provide a range of learning opportunities, and if you are the practice assessor to provide a fair and accurate assessment. All the advice given in earlier chapters around the assessment process applies. As a reminder these are:

- Undertake the initial interview as soon as possible in the first week.
- Look at the feedback from the practice supervisors and practice assessor from the placement where the student failed at the first attempt and at the comments in the ongoing achievement record.
- Identify the elements which were failed and need to be retrieved and agree a clear action plan with SMART objectives to provide the student the best chance to achieve the failed elements.
- Meet regularly and give honest feedback on their progress.
- Ensure regular contact with the Academic Assessor.
- If the student is not meeting the required level of proficiency, seek help from the Academic Assessor/Link Lecturer for you and the student as soon as possible.

Clear and consistent feedback is probably the most essential element in this process as the student will need to be informed of their progress and to be informed early on if they are not making the required progress. As the second attempt is a student's opportunity to demonstrate that they have developed and improved on the first attempt you should have a very clear benchmark to work from. The content and accuracy of the ongoing achievement record will be important as it is this which is used to show student progress and development and areas for improvement. Identify whether the same areas are consistently being picked up on and how those skills/knowledge/behaviours relate to the area the student has failed in their previous placement.

First and Second Attempts Together

Occasionally a student may be trying to retrieve failed elements from the previous year/part of their programme whilst having started the next year/part of their programme. This will usually happen when only a small number of elements are outstanding, and it is not in the student's interest to restrict their progression. This means they may be repeating the outstanding elements from their previous placement in one practice assessment document and being assessed on new elements in the new practice assessment document. This means you will need to be very organised in your role to support and assess this student. Remember, however, that you should have the ongoing achievement record written by the practice assessor of the first attempt placement as a reference point. This should give you a good indicator as to what the student's areas for development and any issues and concerns are. Reflecting on the contents of the ongoing achievement record along with feedback in the practice assessment document with the student will help the development of the action plan for the student.

> ! Discuss the student's development /action plan with the practice supervisors so they can support the student more effectively if there are times when you are not available for the student.

Assessing Multiple Elements in the Practice Assessment Document

In those circumstances where you are being asked to assess the student on elements from their failed first attempt whilst undertaking assessments on new elements in the practice assessment document, your skills of planning for and facilitating learning will come to the fore. You may find it helpful to undertake an initial, midpoint and final interview focussing on the previous failed elements and a separate set of interviews focussing on the new elements. This will help distinguish what is required for each assessment and though a little more documentation is involved it will enable the student to focus on what needs to be done for all areas being assessed. An ongoing achievement record should also be written after a second attempt, regardless of the outcome.

Failing at Second Attempt

If you are supporting a student who has to retrieve elements at a second attempt and they are not making the expected progress it is essential that the Link

Lecturer and Academic Assessor are involved early on so that action plans can be put in place to offer the student the best chance to succeed. Failing at second attempt is discussed further in Chapter 8.

INCIDENTS/ACCIDENTS

Occasionally, unfortunate accidents or incidents do occur in practice in which students may be involved themselves or are a witness to. Needlestick injuries are the most common. However, serious untoward incidents such as an assault by a patient or a patient suicide on a placement are examples which can have a significant impact on a student. For any accident or incident, you will follow the same procedures for the student as you would for any member of staff. Complete both the reporting form used by your organisation and the university reporting form (if they have one). A debrief is essential and so too is letting the Link Lecturer/Academic Assessor know so that they can offer their support to the student in practice.

If the student requires medical intervention and is sent home, the student's placements office should also be informed. When a student has been injured and requires medical intervention, they should be seen by their GP and/or the university occupational health team to make an assessment and decision as to their fitness to return to placement. In some cases, it may be helpful to have a three-way meeting with the student, practice assessor, and Link Lecturer or Academic Assessor, to reflect on the incident to gain a greater insight into what happened and to support the student if they are feeling overwhelmed by the experience.

STUDENTS REQUIRING REASONABLE ADJUSTMENTS

Given that the majority of students are female, you are very likely to find yourself supporting students who are pregnant and so may require adjustments to facilitate their learning on placement. It is also likely that you will be allocated students from time to time with a disability who require reasonable adjustments. Many applicants to nursing cite their own personal experiences as a patient or service user as being one of the main reasons for wanting to become a nurse, so it is not surprising to find that many nursing students identify as having a disability. In 2018–19 15.9% of students who enrolled on nursing courses at university were known to have a disability (HESA, 2019). This includes students with a specific learning difference, a physical disability or impairment or a mental health condition, each of which may require reasonable adjustments to be put in place to support their learning at university and in practice. All students have to be cleared by occupational health as a condition of their entry to the programme but students with a disability, or a physical or mental health condition may require reasonable adjustments to be put in place in order to ensure that they are not disadvantaged. We look at this in more detail in Chapter 10.

Students Who are Pregnant

A risk assessment must be undertaken by the university once a student has disclosed their pregnancy and a pregnancy plan agreed to with regard to any reasonable adjustments they may need, in relation to both the student's academic studies and their placements. The university will need to check with you that the placement is safe for the student. The student will also need to undertake a risk assessment with you before commencing their placement. In completing the risk assessment, you will need to consider what adjustments to the student's activities may be required and the impact on the student's ability to achieve their proficiencies. If following the risk assessment, it is apparent that the student will not be able to undertake a suitable range of practice experiences with you to meet the proficiencies, contact the Link Lecturer or university placement office to discuss. A decision can then be made as to the suitability of another practice area or whether the student may be required to commence their maternity leave earlier than planned. If a pregnant student's health status changes at any point after the risk assessment was completed and she can no longer engage in the learning opportunities available, it will be appropriate to repeat the risk assessment and consider whether further adjustments are required and possible. This will require further discussions with the university.

Reasonable adjustments that may be required for a student who is pregnant will include:

- time off to attend antenatal appointments
- adjustments to shift patterns (later starts if morning sickness is severe, or no night duty)
- extra breaks during a shift.

THE DISINTERESTED STUDENT

Occasionally you may find you have a student placed with you who appears disinterested. There can be many reasons for this. The student may have significant personal problems outside of their placement and course that are impacting on their ability to fully engage and/or causing them mental distress. Alternatively, it may be that the student has particular fears around their placement or is having second thoughts about nursing as a career for them. A significant part of your role is to motivate and encourage students; this may not always be easy because students have different learning styles and what works with one student may not motivate another. Students who are not motivated during a practice placement can be especially challenging. It may be difficult to engage them in placement experiences and they may seem bored or disinterested. A student who is not motivated is unlikely to be learning, so it is important to discover what the problem is and try to re-motivate them as quickly as possible. The following may help to keep you and your students motivated:

- making sure students feel welcomed in your unit/ward/clinic
- give constructive feedback regularly, there are always areas of their practice where you can provide positive feedback when they achieve something or do something well
- make time at the beginning of the shift to ask the student what they wish to learn during the day and ask how you can help them with this
- set realistic goals with the student and ensure any agreed plans are followed
- regularly point out the connection between what the student is doing and the proficiencies or professional values they need to achieve
- if the student does do something incorrectly or unprofessionally address it in a supportive way
- be enthusiastic about your work and avoid being negative about colleagues in the presence of students.

Where a student remains disengaged this needs to be discussed with them and linked to their professional values, which are likely to include engagement with learning opportunities and/or working effectively with others. A discussion with their academic assessor is important as they may be aware of problems the student may be having outside of their placement that you are unaware of. Whilst they may not be able to share this with you without the student's consent, by informing the academic assessor they can explore with the student if these problems are connected and how the student can be supported. They can also ask for permission to share this information with the practice assessor and then have a tripartite meeting with yourself and the student.

STUDENT COMPLAINTS AND RAISING CONCERNS

First, it is important to appreciate the difference between a concern and a complaint raised by a student related to their placement.

- A **complaint** is related to an issue where a student is complaining about how they have personally been treated whilst on a practice education experience and are seeking personal resolution.
- A **concern** relates to something the student has become aware of whilst in the practice setting. It usually relates to an issue, wrongdoing, or risk which affects others and where a person or people may be at risk of harm.

Managing a complaint or a concern raised by a student can be difficult, especially if it relates to one of your colleagues. It can be natural to want to defend them. If a student approaches you with concerns about inappropriate or below-standard care that they have observed or a complaint about how someone has treated them, then take this as a compliment to the relationship you have built with them. It can be very difficult as a student to raise a concern or complaint, as they will be conscious that it may have ramifications for their assessment and how they are viewed by the team they are working with.

Responding to Concerns by a Student

Following his investigation into the events at Mid Staffordshire Hospital NHS Foundation Trust (Francis, 2013) Francis identified that there were problems in the way that staff who raised concerns at the Trust were treated. This led to a further independent review by Francis in which he found that students on placement were particularly vulnerable if they raised concerns (Francis, 2015). Francis found examples of students:

- *'failing' placements after raising concerns when there had previously been no issues regarding their practice*
- *losing placements after raising concerns and ultimately losing their place at university*
- *suffering detriment from co-workers or managers whilst they remained in that placement*

Francis (2015, p. 178)

Research by Brown and Jones (2020) found that the power differential between mentors and students was highly influential on the ability of students to raise concerns with their mentor coupled with the fear of how this might impact on the mentor's assessment decision. An effective relationship was found to be central to a student's ability to raise concerns. The authors suggested that the new role of practice supervisor who was not responsible for making the assessment decision might be more approachable, making it easier for students to raise concerns. Both universities and placement partners have a joint responsibility to ensure that students are aware of the processes for raising concerns and to support them if they do. So, if a student comes to you with a complaint or concern, then first establish exactly what has happened from the student's perspective, what they saw and what was said. This will give you the opportunity to ask clarifying questions and identify if the student is actually raising a complaint or a concern. You will need to be very sensitive in the way you respond to the student. Where possible a representative from the university should also be involved, so that the student is supported. There will be a number of factors that you will need to clarify with the student:

- Has the student genuinely witnessed poor practice, or have they witnessed an intervention that has been poorly explained and therefore they do not fully understand what they observed?
- Is there a personality clash between the student and a member of staff? Has there been any attempt to resolve the conflict?
- Has there been a misunderstanding that has been blown out of proportion?

These questions will help everyone to understand what has happened and ensure no misconceptions have arisen. If it is agreed that the issues raised by the student are a concern (people are at risk of harm) as opposed to a complaint, then the student will need to be informed of the next steps of raising a concern and the investigation process that will follow. At that point a student may decide:

- they wish to go ahead with formally raising the concern
- they wish to raise the concern but to do so anonymously
- they do not wish to raise the concern formally.

The university raising concerns policy will provide guidance on the steps to be followed whichever decision the student makes, and the university will ensure that the student is appropriately supported throughout the process. If people are at risk of immediate harm, then the concerns must be raised as a matter of urgency with the relevant person in your organisation. In this situation statements will need to be collected including from the student who will be supported by the university in writing any statements required and any further meetings held to investigate the concerns raised.

If the issues raised by the student do not fall under either the raising concerns policy or complaints policy, then no further formal action may needed but it is important that the student is debriefed in a tripartite meeting with the practice assessor and Link Lecturer/Academic Assessor so that they are fully supported and understand why the decisions have been made.

> ! Ensure you are familiar with both your organisation's own raising concerns policy and the ones used by the university(ies) who place students with you.

Responding to a Complaint by a Student

If the issues the student raises are identified as a complaint, then steps should be taken locally to try and resolve the issues raised; this may require involving the manager in the placement. If it cannot be easily resolved, then the Link Lecturer/Academic Assessor should be contacted, and an action plan which addresses the issues raised may need to be put in place to support the student. If the issues raised still cannot be resolved, then it may be necessary for the university to raise this with the senior lead for practice in the organisation, and the student may need to use the organisation's own complaints policy.

When the Complaint is About You

The focus so far has been on the student making a complaint about something or someone that does not directly involve you as their practice supervisor or assessor. However, it might happen that the student does complain to the manager or Link Lecturer about your behaviour, actions or lack of action. The less experienced or confident a student is at dealing with conflict the more emotive the complaint may be in its content. This could lead to heated and difficult conversations without effective mediation. The most common cause is around the assessment process or access to wider learning opportunities. Any intervention from the Link Lecturer should mirror what you would do with your student if they came to you with a complaint. The aim is not to apportion blame, rather to establish an understanding of events and agree on a way forward. See this as an opportunity to seek advice and have questions answered to enable you to undertake your role more effectively.

Concerns or Complaints Raised by a Student on an Apprenticeship Programme

If the student is an employee (an apprentice or secondee to the programme) and the concerns or complaints relate to a placement in their own organisation, then the organisation's own policies and procedures must be followed but the university must also be informed.

WHEN PATIENTS OR SERVICE USERS REFUSE CARE FROM STUDENTS

More often than not patients, service users, carers and families do not object to students being present as an observer or participant in their care. Occasionally, patients will decline permission for students to be present or you might exercise your professional judgement and ask the student not to join you in a certain care activity/interaction. This can be frustrating for the student. However, the NMC are very clear that universities and their practice learning partners must:

> *ensure people have the opportunity to give and if required, withdraw, their informed consent to students being involved in their care*

NMC (2018e, p. 6)

The challenge then is helping students learn about the assessment and interventions you would be performing with the patient or service user. They may also need to be helped to understand why somebody might say 'no' and why decisions may need to be made to exclude students from participating in some care activities.

Here are a few suggestions of what you can do with your student on those occasions when they cannot participate in the care delivery process.

- Ask the student to review the patient's notes to look for indicators of why the patient may decline a student presence.
- Ask the student to review the patient's notes and care plans and identify where the specific assessment or intervention they are not able to participate in, fits into the overall care plan.

- Ask the student to research the evidence base and organisation's policies for the assessment or intervention you will be using – the student could do a presentation to you afterwards.
- Ask the student to engage in an activity which supports the intervention: for example preparation of the trolley and equipment ready for a wound dressing; calculating the drug dosage of an injection.
- Role play the assessment or intervention to be performed and encourage reflection in action to highlight how personal space could be invaded, how exposing this can feel for the individual and how personal the intervention may be.

Using activities such as this allow the student to learn about the specific assessment or intervention, participate at a distance and not feel wholly excluded. They can also help them understand the patient experience. By allocating the student a learning activity for the time you are with the patient, you have planned a learning experience and are indirectly supervising and supporting them. This can alleviate feelings of frustration for the student at not being able to participate.

THE PRESSURES OF SUPERVISING AND ASSESSING STUDENTS

Supporting students on a regular basis can be quite demanding. It can become difficult when problems arise during their placement and the student needs more time to supervise them, more time to provide feedback and potentially more meetings with the student and link lecturers or academic assessors. Time is a precious resource in practice, and you may find it difficult to balance the needs of the patient with the needs of the student. Additional pressures may include supporting the failing student, making the decision to fail a student, and staff shortages. The NMC SSSA standards make clear that both practice supervisors and practice assessors should receive ongoing support in order to fulfil their role (NMC, 2018b). Group meetings within your place of work to share the highs and lows can be a valuable source of peer support and also provide you with opportunities to hear about best practice that you can adopt as well as sharing what has worked for you. When it is particularly busy or there are staff shortages acknowledging this with the students at the start of the shift is important. Consider sharing responsibilities for students across the team (including other healthcare professionals) and inform the students that there will be an opportunity later in the day to meet up as a group, review learning from the day and answer questions they may have. Alternatively, allocating junior students to senior students with the promise to undertake a reflective review before the end of the shift to explore the senior student's experience of supervising a junior student can all be approaches that can ensure the students' learning needs are met whilst ensuring the needs of patients are also met.

THE SUPPORT AVAILABLE TO YOU

Whatever the challenges you face in supporting students in practice there are a range of resources available to help you. Always seek help if you are unsure what to do or are faced with a situation about which you have limited knowledge or experience, or the situation has posed additional challenges for you or the student. Resources available to you are:

- other practice supervisors or practice assessors in your workplace
- the manager in the placement
- the academic assessor
- The link lecturer
- the clinical placement facilitator
- the lead for practice in your organisation
- practice educators/lecturer practitioners
- university handbooks for practice supervisors/assessors
- the university website/placement website
- the NMC website *Supporting information on standards for student supervision and assessment.*

CHALLENGES WHEN THE STUDENT IS AN APPRENTICE

All apprentices are employees and therefore any concerns related to apprentices may require their employer to be informed as well as the university. This relates to issues or concerns related to:

- Attendance, sickness and absence
- Non-compliance with shifts
- Incidents or accidents
- Significant life events where this is impacting their performance. You should discuss with the student about sharing information with their employer and encourage them to discuss with their employer so they can support them.
- Implementing reasonable adjustments particularly where additional equipment may be required.
- Any concerns or complaints raised by the student or against the student.

Action Points

- Make sure you have copies of the university policies relevant to students on practice placements or know where they can be accessed.
- Find time to reflect on the way you handle any challenges with a student and how you might respond to a similar situation next time (record this for your next revalidation with the NMC).
- Seek out and share ideas for managing the student learning experience with colleagues on other placements.
- Ensure you know the contact details of the Link Lecturer and the Academic Assessor so that you can seek advice if you are unsure how to respond to difficult or challenging situations involving a student.
- Arrange to meet with your Freedom to Speak Up Guardian to understand their role and how raising concerns are managed in your organisation.

Chapter 12

Using Simulated Learning

Chapter Outline

INTRODUCTION

Simulated learning in healthcare programmes has developed significantly in recent years and is used widely in both universities and hospitals. Today, it encompasses a wide range of approaches from traditional skills teaching to virtual simulations. The purpose of this chapter is to gain insight into how simulation can be used in pre-registration nurse education in clinical practice as well as at the university. Highly popular with students, simulation provides

A Nurse's Survival Guide to Supervising and Assessing. https://doi.org/10.1016/B978-0-7020-8147-7.00012-0

students with the opportunity to learn skills and make mistakes within a safe environment. This chapter will look at the strategies for planning a simulation and selecting the best type of simulation for the required learning to take place. For successful simulated learning, preparation of self, colleagues, role players and students is essential. The process for this will be discussed, providing examples of simulation briefs for participants. An essential part of any teaching is feedback, but in simulation the use of debriefing following simulation is also essential, enabling the student to reflect on and learn from the simulation experience.

WHAT IS SIMULATED LEARNING?

Simulated learning has a long history in nursing. In the early years the focus was primarily on psychomotor skills – for example, teaching clinical skills such as bed-making and clinical observations. Today it is widely used in pre-registration nursing, midwifery, medical and allied health programmes and has expanded its repertoire to include many of the softer skills around therapeutic engagement with patients and service users, with a significant increase in the use of technology to enhance the student experience. In addition, we are now seeing an increase in field-specific simulation. A quick search of the literature will identify examples of simulated learning related to children's nursing (Gamble, 2017; Wyllie & Batley, 2019), mental health nursing (Felton & Wright, 2017) and learning disability nursing (Saunder & Knight, 2017).

In all aspects of healthcare, there is an increased focus on patient safety and quality indicators. Simulation-based education can help practitioners at all levels to reduce risk and improve the safety and quality of patient care. You may feel this is only relevant to lecturers in the university but as this chapter will show, simulation can be used and indeed is increasingly being used, in healthcare organisations for the education and training of their staff. With the new Nursing and Midwifery Council (NMC) standards for nursing it also offers practice supervisors and assessors in practice alternative opportunities to enable their students to achieve the new NMC proficiencies (NMC, 2018d). In addition, universities are keen to increase involvement of clinical staff in university simulation centres, with the NMC seeing this as best practice. Simulated learning is also important because simulation hours undertaken at university can count towards the 2300 hours students are required to achieve by the end of their programme. The NMC no longer specifies an upper limit to the number of hours of simulated learning that can count towards these 2300 hours; only that it should address specific learning or clinical needs and for adult nursing students must comply with the European Directive 2005/36/EC in the approach used for simulating clinical learning.

First, don't be daunted. Simulation is simply another tool in your repertoire of teaching and learning skills and although it may include technologically advanced tools, it doesn't have to. The NMC (2018c, p.18) defines simulation as:

an artificial representation of a real world practice scenario that supports student development through experiential learning with the opportunity for repetition, feedback, evaluation and reflection. Effective simulation facilitates safety by enhancing knowledge, behaviours and skills.

Students are required to respond to situations in simulations as they would in the clinical environment, usually in real time, applying and integrating knowledge skills and critical thinking. Preparation for, debriefing from, and feedback on performance are crucial to the process to ensure that learning is accompanied by assessment (usually informal) and reinforcement of good practice. Participants are active rather than passive receivers of information. This 'learning by doing' approach is one that suits many nursing students.

WHY USE SIMULATION?

Simulation is used in many disciplines, particularly when the reality may be dangerous, events are rare, and/or errors are costly in human and/or financial terms. Obvious examples are the aviation industry, where sophisticated flight simulators are mandatory in the training of pilots to maintain their skills; the military; and in the nuclear power industry. Although the use of simulation and simulators has a relatively long history in medical and nursing education, the NMC has increasingly recognised simulation as an essential component of nursing and midwifery programmes (NMC, 2018c). The use of skills and simulation enables students to build self-confidence by providing the opportunity for them to acquire, develop and refine clinical skills in an environment which is both safe and supportive. It encourages hands-on thinking, developing decision-making, communication, dexterity and critical thinking to acquire a holistic approach to care delivery.

USING SIMULATION IN NURSE EDUCATION

Students on nursing programmes need to learn practical clinical skills and therapeutic communication skills in order to develop the level of proficiency set out in the NMC's *Standards of proficiency for registered nurses* NMC (2018d). Some of these psychomotor skills are technically advanced; in the wider context of patient care, many involve high levels of cognition, critical thinking and communication skills. It would appear that the acquisition and development of competence in these skills is becoming more challenging as the complexity of healthcare increases and the context changes. As modes of healthcare delivery change, there may be fewer opportunities for students to experience certain aspects of care or practise specific skills during their placements. This has become more apparent with the increasing move to telemedicine and reduced length of patient stay in hospitals.

NMC Standards of Proficiency

The new NMC *Standards of proficiency for registered nurses* (NMC, 2018d) have meant a radical rethink about the use of simulation for nurses by both universities and placement providers. The Standards include two annexes:

- Annexe A: Communication and relationship management skills
- Annexe B: Nursing procedures

The new proficiencies apply to ALL four fields of practice and yet many are commonly viewed as only available to specific fields of practice. As a consequence, some of the skills in these two annexes have caused concerns for both universities and placement providers as being challenging to be achieved across all fields. The NMC (2018d) acknowledges this challenge and notes that each field will develop differing levels of expertise and knowledge with respect to some of the skills in the annexes, specifically identifying:

- Annexe A, Section 3: Evidence-based, best-practice communication skills and approaches for providing therapeutic interventions and
- Annexe B, Part I: Procedures for assessing needs for person-centred care, sections 1 and 2.

These annexes can be found in Appendix 1 at the end of this book. However, the NMC expects that all students regardless of field will have achieved sufficient proficiency in them relative to their field of practice. This is where simulation, be it in the real world of practice or at the university, offers an alternative way of achieving these proficiencies.

> ! Look at the annexes in Appendix 1 and consider which of the proficiencies you can offer in your placement and which may prove more of a challenge for a student to achieve.

Students now gain experience in a variety of settings other than inpatient care. Whilst this is entirely appropriate, it means that students' exposure to the hospital environment, where many clinical skills were traditionally honed, is reduced. Even in the hospital setting, changing practices – for example, the increase in day case surgery – mean that students may not have the opportunity to practise certain skills, such as suture removal, now frequently done in the community after discharge. Practice staff have many competing demands upon their time, whilst the NMC *Code* (2018a) requires all qualified nurses to support students, the needs of patients will by necessity take priority. However, including students when new learning opportunities arise is essential if they are to develop the proficiencies you will want them to have when they qualify and join you as a registered nurse.

Against this background of an increasing patient safety and risk manage-ment agenda and reduced availability of traditional clinical placements, the interest in and demand for simulation-based training has increased. Simulation is being recognised as a way of offering the opportunity to train multi-professional groups of staff for real patient situations in a realistic context in a way that is risk-free for patients and, if correctly facilitated, risk-free for staff. Through simulation-based teaching, students are provided with the opportunity to rehearse skills, procedures and events not often used. They are also provided with an opportunity to refine and develop skills used on a more frequent basis but which cannot be rehearsed and practised in the real environment for practi-cal and/or ethical reasons.

SIMULATION IN CLINICAL PRACTICE

Healthcare organisations have invested in a range of approaches to simulated learning, including high- and low-fidelity manikins, skill stations, task train-ers, workshops, role play and virtual reality simulations, which are increasingly involving multi-professional groups. Often, they make use of a vacant space such as a side room or empty ward area; many organisations now have dedicated skills centres. These have the advantage of creating a more realistic environment and it is an alternative approach that can be used by practice supervisors/assessors. It is likely therefore that you are already familiar with many of these approaches.

In either setting, the key to a successful learning experience is an enthusias-tic, able and clinically credible facilitator.

PROVISION OF SIMULATED LEARNING

There are many ways to provide simulation-based training. Sometimes simula-tion will involve highly sophisticated manikins; at other times it may involve actors or a mixture of both. Simulated learning can also take place in a virtual environment in the form of interactive computer-based learning packages.

The key to all of these approaches is *immersion*. The scenario or patient situation created must be as realistic as possible in order that the participant becomes immersed in it and reacts and responds as if it were real. Simulation most often takes place in a university-based setting where students and practitio-ners come together to provide this experience with the support of the students' lecturers. Whilst these facilities are often well equipped and provide access to staff who are experienced in simulation, it requires a high level of planning and coordination to get everyone in the same place at the same time.

CHOOSING THE BEST TYPE OF SIMULATION

The type of simulation chosen for any particular learning experience will be dic-tated by the learning outcomes and facilities available and so must be carefully thought through beforehand. Harder (2010) undertook a systematic review of three key types of simulation:

- low-fidelity, involving simulated situations, task trainers or non-computerised simulation methods
- mid-fidelity, involving the use of standardised/simulated patients
- high-fidelity simulation, which uses computerised human patient simulator manikins.

However, today we can also add:

- virtual reality, computer-based and online simulation.

The following sections provide some examples of simulated scenarios you may like to be involved in or could use in your workplace or in a skills/simulation centre.

Role Play and Actors

A simulated clinical scenario can be created with people acting as the patient/service user, and/or in some cases a relative. The 'actors' may be professional actors or a standardised patient (SP). SPs are usually volunteers who have been prepared for various roles. More usually the 'actors' will be colleagues; ideally, they should not be someone with whom the student is very familiar. It is very difficult for the student to relate to someone as a patient when they are in fact known to them, such as the ward sister or a university lecturer, and this detracts from the realism of the learning experience. Preparation of the actor, whether they be professionals, SPs or colleagues, is essential. They need to be clear about the student's learning outcomes and avoid any tendency to overact or ad lib. You may like to consider giving them a detailed synopsis of who they are, perhaps even based on a 'real' patient they can identify with. This will be easier if they are not known to the student. When using actors one of the key learning objectives is usually related to communication skills, and the 'patient' can be primed to exhibit certain behaviours or ask particular questions but should react as realistically as possible to what the student actually does or says. Importantly, they can also provide feedback to the student on how well they communicated and undertook the care activities.

Role players/actors are particularly valuable for simulations where the focus is on therapeutic communication skills, and they are increasingly used for mental health students in universities. The involvement of children or people with a learning disability in simulations is more problematic, as it requires consideration of issues around safeguarding and management of consent.

Most universities and some healthcare organisations have a bank of patients/service users who have been prepared to participate in simulations with staff and healthcare students and are a valuable resource in making the experience 'real' for students. Students also appreciate and take the feedback provided by them more seriously.

> ! If you use actors during a simulation exercise, then it is essential to prepare them beforehand on how to stay in character.

Mixed Task Trainer/Actor

Using this approach an actor can be used in conjunction with a training manikin or task trainer such as a catheterisation model or venipuncture/cannulation arm. This allows the student to practise a potentially hazardous technique safely but in the context of a patient situation.

An example of a possible scenario is as follows:

A student is asked to give care to a patient who has diabetes and requires a subcutaneous injection of insulin. An actor is briefed for the role and informed that they are newly diagnosed with diabetes and will be dressed in a hospital gown, sitting in a chair. An injectable pad is taped to the actor so that the student can demonstrate their injection technique. The lecturer practice supervisor/assessor will observe from the side so that they can see and hear what takes place. The student will be expected to demonstrate that they can give the medication correctly, communicate with the patient, answer questions and explain exactly what they are doing. At the end of the simulation the student will receive feedback as part of a debriefing to ensure they are clear about what they did well and areas for future development.

Alternatively, a student could be required to simulate a catheterisation technique by communicating with an actor but performing the actual task on a catheterisation model. The learning activity would require the student to demonstrate the following:

- Correct checking and preparation of all equipment.
- Gaining the patient's consent and providing adequate explanation.
- Answer the patient questions knowledgeably and in a way that will help to allay anxiety.
- Recognise if at any point further assistance is needed.
- Demonstrate safe and effective catheterisation technique.

Use of Patient Simulators

There are many patient simulators on the market, some highly sophisticated and capable of producing highly realistic physiological responses that might be exhibited by a patient in a variety of states of health and illness (high fidelity simulators). These are best suited to creating a scenario where the main objective is for the students to assess, observe, interpret and act on physiological changes that cannot be recreated in an actor. The addition of a 'patient voice' to the manikin enables the students to verbally interact with the patient. For example, a patient simulator can be set up as a postoperative patient (intravenous fluids running, catheter, wounds, drains and dressing in situ, oxygen in place). The patient simulator can be used to recreate signs of shock due to blood loss.

This kind of simulation can be resource intensive; someone is needed to operate the simulator and voice. This could be, but is not necessarily, the same person. In many cases it is helpful to have someone other than the person facilitating the simulation to be the person who is called upon to help. The more realistic you can make the simulation the better the learning experience for the student. If you are undertaking a simulation exercise in practice, consider having the actual person involved (e.g. the senior nurse or colleague who would be called in a real-life situation), as this makes it all the more real. In addition to this, you may choose to have other actors taking on other roles, for example as other patients or relatives who are either present or on the telephone.

In a scenario with an acutely ill adult or child, the student must demonstrate:

- Full systematic ABCDE assessment of the patient/child
- Interpret and act upon the findings of the assessment appropriately
- Document findings and seek appropriate help
- Communicate with the patient/child and/or relative throughout in a manner that is knowledgeable and reassuring
- Provide a clear, concise and relevant handover using Situation, Background, Assessment, Recommendation (SBAR) to the relevant member of staff.

All these examples of simulated experiences allow students to practise their skills and apply knowledge to patient care in a realistic and contextualised way. This approach can prepare them for similar situations in the real world of practice. This also allows assessment of and feedback on skills and knowledge in a way that is risk-free to patients and the student.

Virtual Reality, Computer-based and Online Simulation

This includes virtual worlds, virtual environments, virtual patients, virtual reality task trainers, and serious games (Cant et al., 2019). There are a wide range of online resources which can be used before or after immersive simulation experiences, to enhance the acquisition of skills and to explore the evidence underpinning practice and so integrating theory and practice. Examples available in the UK are:

- Laerdal vSim for nursing
- Oxford Medical Simulation (OMS)

There are also an increasing number of sophisticated virtual reality simulations available. These may utilise virtual reality headsets or a simple computer screen. The virtual worlds created here are similar to online video games. The student enters the virtual world and can move around within it, assessing and responding to virtual patients carrying out tasks and making decisions, all in real time with built-in feedback. These virtual reality simulations can be used as part of e-learning, can be undertaken at a time of the student's choosing, and do not require the intervention of a facilitator.

Covid-19 has accelerated the use of online simulations, which occur live in real time, often using actors with whom students interact. These simulations can replicate online assessments or consultations that many healthcare professionals are now having with patients and require planning facilitation and debriefing.

In addition, computer-based learning modules, whilst they do not simulate the real world, enable students to learn at their own pace and use real world scenarios, for example:

- *Safe Medicate*, to support the development and assessment of competent practice in medication administration.
- *Clinicalskills.net* which has over 250 guidelines of clinical skills procedures.
- *E-learning for Healthcare* widely used by the NHS and which has a range of on-line modules.

ARE YOU AND YOUR AREA PREPARED FOR SIMULATED LEARNING?

Before you start to use simulation within your role in supporting students, whether in the clinical area or in an educational establishment, you must ensure that you have prepared both yourself and the learning environment.

IDENTIFYING OPPORTUNITIES FOR SIMULATION

You should start by asking yourself why you would like to use simulation as an approach to learning. Some key questions include:

- What aspects of practice learning will we be using simulation for?
- Why is simulation useful here?
- What is the outcome or level of practice activity that we want the student to perform?

No doubt you will be able to identify a number quite quickly. For example, simulation is easily adaptable and a great learning experience for the following types of situations:

- patient assessment
- key clinical skills and procedures
- communication skills, both core skills and advanced skills such as de-escalation strategies and techniques
- basic and advanced life support.

When planning a session, you need to consider the following:

- How many students will you have?

- Where is the simulation taking place? In the trust/clinical area or in an educational establishment?
- What are the learning outcomes to be achieved?
- What behaviours/actions are you expecting from students as part of the session?
- If some students are observing – what else will they be doing at that time?
- What resources do you have, and which other staff are available to help?

PLANNING EFFECTIVE SIMULATION

The simulated learning environment needs to be as realistic as possible, so what is learnt and rehearsed is transferred easily into future practice. Within clinical areas it may be relatively easy to recreate a realistic environment as equipment and appropriate resources will be readily available. Empty wards and clinical areas are ideal venues for simulation as they can be quickly transformed into a realistic clinical environment and many healthcare organisations now have purpose-built teaching wards and simulation suites.

Within a university, simulation will require careful planning and sufficient resources to 'mock up' a convincing clinical setting. Planning will need to start early, so that equipment and supplies are available in good time.

On any manikin or human actor used within the simulation a range of recipes and procedures can be incorporated to mimic appropriate clinical situations or conditions such as bleeding, fake vomit, malaena, pus, etc. This practice is often referred to in the literature and simulator user guides as 'moulage'. The internet is a valuable resource for tips and useful recipes for 'moulage'.

! If using a closed ward or side room ensure that clear notices are put on all entry doors to ensure that real staff, patients and visitors within the organisation do not wander in unexpectedly.

Preparing Teaching/Clinical Colleagues

Before commencing the simulation session, you should discuss and agree both the learning outcomes and the session with any other colleagues who will be involved. During this discussion it is important that any constraints or concerns are acknowledged and that there is a realistic approach to what can be achieved in the session. Discuss and agree how time will be distributed throughout the session, ensuring that there is enough time for debriefing at the end, as this is where much of the learning takes place. Outline the learning resources/material (i.e. patient histories/scripts, etc. that will be required for the simulation) and agree who will be preparing this ahead of the session. Ensure all clinical/

teaching staff involved are familiar with the plan, environment and equipment prior to the session. Having a trial run without students is very useful and supportive for those staff new to simulation, if there is time.

> ! When planning your first simulation exercise try to keep it simple and of short duration. This will minimise the amount of planning and organisation required and allows you to build slowly upon success without becoming disheartened.

Preparing the Students

In order for the simulation session to have the maximum impact on student learning, it is important to ensure that students are prepared. Information can be made available regarding the scenario/patient and associated practice issues ahead of the session. This will ensure that students can prepare for the session by reviewing appropriate theory and practice guidelines and that they have some idea what will be expected of them during the simulation. If high-fidelity simulators are being used as part of the session, time must be allocated prior to the simulation to familiarise students with what the simulator can and cannot do, so that they know how to relate to it once it becomes 'their patient'.

Using a Simulation Planning Tool

To ensure that all aspects of the planning are adequately addressed prior to the session it is useful to have a planning tool template that all staff involved in simulation can refer to or use. An example of this is provided in Box 12.1. Clear objectives or learning outcomes are essential so both you and the students know what the simulation is trying to achieve (see appendix 1 at the end of this chapter). Consider the following headings in determining what you want the student to achieve:

- knowledge they need to gain/show
- skills to be performed
- satisfaction by participants including role players
- demonstration of critical thinking and problem-solving skills
- self confidence.

You may find the student's practice assessment document will give you some ideas for possible objectives or learning outcomes.

Preparation of Students Prior to Session

Before you can commence a simulated learning activity you will need to check that students have completed the necessary tutorials or online programmes related to the topic area, if available, or point them to key policies or guidelines.

BOX 12.1 Template/Checklist for Designing a Simulation Session

Date/Time of Session:	Title of Session:
Number of Students:	

Learning outcomes for session:

Simulation scenario which would provide the desired physiology/Outline of storyboard

Identify resources needed/provided – time/staff, equipment, expertise?

Supporting material required/suggested	Provided?
Storyboard for students ahead of session – can be posted on virtual learning environment or in a teaching pack	Yes/No
Facilitator's notes, including a full version of the scenario and the behaviours/responses/actions you expect of the students	Yes/No
Information for the 'patient', whether that is the person providing the voice of the simulator, or the 'actor' who will be the patient	Yes/No
A full equipment list and, if using the simulators, information on the scenario needed	Yes/No
A checklist related to student behaviour/actions/responses expected	Yes/No
Activity identified for students waiting their turn for simulation	Yes/No
Time allocated format for debriefing/feedback	Yes/No
Students provided with a reflection/action plan sheet for inclusion in their portfolio	Yes/No
Evaluation tool developed/included	Yes/No

For example, when creating a simulated subcutaneous injection exercise, you should ensure students have prior knowledge of:

● subcutaneous injection technique
● infection control
● hand washing
● drug administration
● health and safety in practice (e.g. disposal of sharps).

At the start of the session, ground rules will need to be agreed within the group – these may include aspects such as:

● constructively and positively supporting each other during the simulation
● focusing on the performance not the person when giving feedback
● agreeing whether the facilitator can be asked for information during the simulation

● agreeing whether students can ask for 'time out/pause' if they want to stop the simulation.

Having ground rules such as these will encourage students to feel less anxious during the simulation, so that they can view it as a learning opportunity rather than an 'examination'. Students will also benefit from having a very clear scenario to work from as this will provide the necessary background from which they will enter the simulation event.

Information for Role Players

If you are going to use role players in a simulation exercise, then it is very important for them to understand their role and what is expected of them during the activity. For example, they may need to 'act' a certain way: angry, anxious, in pain, confused. Any actor involved in simulation will need some clear instructions on the types of behaviour they might need to display and also some background about past health history and current health state. The type of information that an actor for the scenario described earlier may require will fall under a minimum of four key headings:

■ Past medical history, for example:
  ● 'You have recently been diagnosed as a diabetic – you are struggling to control the diabetes with your diet.'
■ History of your present illness, for example:
  ● 'You collapsed while playing football. You have not eaten since a curry late last night and you had a few beers.'
■ Behaviour, for example:
  ● You don't like doctors or hospital
  ● You feel 'awful' and don't want to be 'messed around'
  ● You are very impatient and just want to get home
  ● You wince loudly when the injection is given – and shout out 'is that your first time!'
■ Questions and prompts, for example:
  ● Answer student questions but show you are irritated by them
  ● Ask why you need the injection
  ● Be defensive when answering any questions about your lifestyle and diet

FEEDBACK FORMS

During the simulation sessions, it is helpful to complete a feedback sheet which identifies the range of student behaviours expected. This form should include assessment of aspects of communication skills, professional behaviour, technical skills and health and safety considerations.

In addition, it is useful for the simulated patient/actor to provide feedback on how they felt the student did, especially commenting on their communication skills. This makes the role of simulated patient much more meaningful for the actor and can be a way of ensuring service user input into healthcare curricula and student assessment. All of the feedback can be incorporated into 'the debrief' which follows the simulation.

> ! It is useful for the actors within a simulation to deliver feedback while they are in character. Actors should be prepared for how to give this feedback, for example, how to respond to both good and poor practice.

When organising a simulated learning exercise, you will want it to run smoothly with no major problems and difficulties. If you plan well for the event, then there is a good chance that it will run according to plan. However, the reality is that sometimes it is the opposite of this that actually takes place. It's a good idea therefore to identify what potential problems might occur during a simulated learning exercise so systems can be put in place to prevent problems before they arise.

Poor preparation for a simulation session can cause confusion, frustration and dissatisfaction for everyone involved. It is essential to have clear goals, so everyone is clear what is to be achieved This requires adequate preparation of the simulation, clear objectives and learning outcomes and guidance for students, role players, technicians and all staff involved. Initially your simulation session/experience may not be perfect; however, you should strive to create a positive learning experience and environment for the students involved. You will need to put some time and effort into planning the simulation exercise to ensure that it runs smoothly and it feels as 'real' as possible.

PERSONAL PREPARATION

Assuming that you work in a clinical area that is suitable for running simulations, the next step is to ensure that you are personally prepared for your role as a facilitator.

What Skills Do You Need to Facilitate Learning?

In facilitation, the emphasis moves from teacher-centred to student-centred learning. As a facilitator your role is in enabling and encouraging the student to discover what they need to know and guiding them to the acquisition of that knowledge rather than knowing it all yourself. This can be quite challenging, but what is more important is the relationship between the student and the facilitator, which allows the student to feel comfortable and able to make mistakes safely and without ridicule.

If doing this with a group you need to consider group dynamics and create an atmosphere that promotes and allows safety, trust, enjoyment, listening, sharing and even non-participation, which are all important elements of effective facilitation. Valuing and sharing the contributions of students will encourage participation and therefore promote learning.

Preparation for your role as a facilitator and gaining further experience is important. You may have covered facilitation skills during workshops to prepare you as a practice supervisor or assessor or coach or by undertaking a teaching course. Having completed preparation for your role, it is useful to take the opportunity to observe or assist with a simulation session to develop and refine your skills as part of your own professional development within a safe environment. Even experienced teachers with many hours of facilitation are expected to engage in peer review of their teaching practice to help them hone their skill. As facilitation can be considered as quite a demanding and intense process, leading to occasional discomfort, anxiety and insecurity, preparation and support for the role is crucial to the creation of a successful learning environment. If there is insufficient preparation for your role and a lack of opportunity to reflect on the effectiveness of your facilitation skills, this can result in an awkward teaching session that is little more than a string of orchestrated techniques. Some trusts/clinical areas encourage staff to participate in simulation activities either within the Trust or at the local university. In other areas this is taken further, with the opportunity to attend 'train the trainer' programmes related to the use of simulation.

The opportunity for you to develop your facilitation skills through supporting a simulation session will allow you to 'grow and develop' as a practitioner at the same time as supporting the 'growth and development' of the students you come into contact with. While the actual simulation experience is a valuable learning opportunity, the real growth and development will come through your own preparation for the simulation and then reflection on your strengths and identification of areas for future development as a facilitator.

> ! Consider a 'mock' simulation exercise with your colleagues before inviting students to take part. This should iron out any practical issues such as availability of resources and the role of actors.

If specific training on simulation is not available in your area, take the opportunity to find out what your students are doing at the university. Find out what simulation scenarios are part of their programme and help prepare and maintain student resources in your area to support this learning. If you get the chance, go and observe simulation taking place at work or in the local university and once you feel confident ask to take part.

DEBRIEFING AS PART OF SIMULATION

Discussion after the simulation is an important aspect of the learning process, and an essential element of learning involving simulation. Debriefing requires reflection on action and enables students to grow professionally and transfer their learning to future practice.

For this reason, debriefing after simulation should never be treated as dispensable or unnecessary. Kolbe et al. (2015) explore approaches to debriefing and the dilemmas of judgemental and non-judgemental debriefing.

They advocate the importance of discussing mistakes made in a supportive way to enable a positive learning experience. The purpose of debriefing after simulation is to:

- Enable the student to reflect on and analyse their actions.
- Assist the student to evaluate their own performance.
- Assist the student to evaluate their understanding of the clinical situation.
- Assist the student to evaluate how to improve their practice.

Before the simulation exercise you should have taken time to personally prepare yourself and the student for the simulation, identifying and reinforcing learning outcomes. The same consideration needs to be given to where, how and when you will debrief.

Ideally debriefing occurs immediately after the simulation. If you are unable to guarantee free uninterrupted time immediately after the simulation exercise you should identify a time to meet as soon as possible after. It is essential that you gain the trust of your student early in your relationship, as you will rely on this for the debriefing to be valued. Debriefing is a student-centred activity but is facilitator-led. The approach is best thought of as a guided reflection to enabling students to explore emotions, thoughts, impressions and reactions, as well as reviewing facts, and receiving and giving feedback.

There are many different models of debriefing, which include: Three Phase (Rudolf et al., 2006) 3-D (Zigmont et al., 2011) Gather, Analyse, Summarise (GAS) (Burke & Mancuso, 2012) The Diamond (Jaye et al., 2015). You may well choose elements of several in developing your own approach or base your approach on a model of reflection with which you feel comfortable, for example Gibbs (1988) model of reflection (Fig. 12.1).

Debriefing after a simulation exercise will provide an opportunity to practise your active listening skills. Beware that your own views, feelings and opinions do not dominate. You will need to indicate that you are interested and reinforce the value of the student's views and opinions.

Whilst debriefing focuses primarily on the student and their reflections, guided by the facilitator, and is usually formative or developmental, it may well be appropriate as described above to include aspects of feedback. Feedback is different to debriefing; it is teacher-centred and involves the facilitator, the simulated patient and/or other students providing information to the student, often against pre-set criteria or standards of practice (Fig. 12.2)

Whilst this is not essential, debriefing and feedback may be further enhanced by the use of video recordings of the simulation, which can be played back. Students must always be made aware if the simulations are being recorded and the purpose and use of the recording made clear, as well as assurance as to how the recording will be used or destroyed following the simulation. Discussion on this is often part of the ground rules agreed at the start. If the recording is to be used for a future purpose – for example, educational sessions or conference

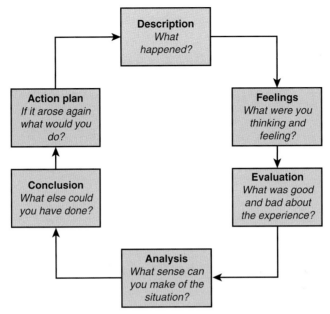

FIG. 12.1   Model of reflection. *(From Gibbs (1988) with kind permission of OCSLD, Oxford Brookes University.)*

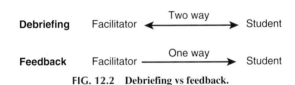

FIG. 12.2   Debriefing vs feedback.

presentations – informed and written consent from all those involved should be obtained.

Playing back recorded elements of simulations can be very useful in reinforcing good practice or the achievement of learning outcomes when these have been demonstrated by a student. Very cautious use is advised when playing back elements that were less positive, as this can be humiliating and counterproductive to learning but may have a place when a very safe and trusting learning environment has been created.

PLANNING FOR THE DEBRIEF

You should never undertake a simulation exercise until you have clearly thought about the learning outcomes and the behaviours and actions the student is required to demonstrate. For the feedback element it is useful to design a simple tick sheet that outlines the various areas in which you want the student to develop with areas for comment and short notes (Box 12.2). You can then use

BOX 12.2 Example Feedback Sheet

Simulation Feedback Sheet for a Post-operative Patient
Student name:
Date:

Expected Behaviours	0	1	2	3	4	5	Comment
Personal professional presentation							
Applies alcohol gel/washes hands at appropriate times							
Communicates and assesses level of patient consciousness and pain							
Systematically assesses vital signs and fluid balance							
Observes wound sites							
Interprets vital signs correctly							
Documents/ charts information accurately							
Communicates findings							
Demonstrates/discusses basic knowledge and understanding of the importance of post-operative observations							

What did the student do well?
Areas for the student to focus on for the future:
General comments:
Signed:
Name:

these comments and notes as a basis for any feedback provided as part of 'the debrief' after the session. Your feedback should take account of specific client care demonstrated in the simulation and the student's stage of learning.

You may be able to ask the student or group of students to use the tick/comment sheet on each other. This can be a powerful way to develop reflective skills and contribute to effective feedback; however, you will need to remember that some aspects of peer assessment can provoke anxiety if the peer group are close working colleagues or friends. Here, your knowledge of the students will help.

The decision of how you would like to design debriefing following simulation is clearly in your hands. You should always remember that there is a tension between making the student responsible for their own learning and ensuring achievement of specific learning objectives. Your understanding of the learning that must be met underpins all preparation. Certainly, simulation undertaken within a course should show specifically identified intended learning outcomes; in practice placements you can use the practice assessment document for the appropriate learning outcomes. This should mean that the student is aware of what they should be learning and be making a plan as to how they will do this, under your guidance and expertise. As a general rule the debriefing element should comprise at least two-thirds of the total session time.

Structuring the Debrief

Phases of debriefing which are common to many of the models are:

Reactions

Here as the facilitator you can guide the reflection and discussion by encouraging the students to verbalise their emotional response, and then review the facts within a respectful and supportive environment. Thoughtful discussion allows the student to sort out events and interpret what happened and why. Sometimes a student will lack insight into their capabilities, and therefore feedback can be provided at this point in order to reinforce their self-confidence. Listening and responding to what the students say is crucial, as is acknowledging the aspects that are important to them, which may not be the same as yours.

Analysis

Explore the experience as it relates to the learning outcomes. Listen and use silence to promote reflection and discussion and express empathy and acceptance as appropriate. Provide feedback regarding the achievement of learning outcomes and encourage feedback and comment from peers and/or simulated patients if relevant.

Thoughtful discussion allows the student to sort out events and interpret what happened and why. Analysing and exploring provides the opportunity for new understanding and generalisation from this experience to practice.

Summary

At this point revisit and review what has been discussed and were there any common themes that emerged? Ask the students what learning they will take away from the session. In addition, you as the facilitator may have learnt as a result of the session and you could consider sharing this with the students.

The key objective of 'the debrief' is to enhance critical thinking and problem solving, enabling the student to learn from their successes and identify the areas that require improvement or development. This type of reflection will show you if the student has insight into their own abilities, and how they might progress and develop their skills.

Always try to be constructive. You may need to help students identify a progression plan, which includes areas the student can work on to improve, progress and develop. While some students will have ideas on how to develop themselves, others who are less experienced or confident will rely on you for guidance and advice.

EVALUATING THE SIMULATION

It is important to evaluate the effectiveness of the simulation afterwards. You could develop a short survey for the student(s) to complete. Explain that part of their professional development as a nurse is developing the ability to provide constructive honest feedback, as many students may find it difficult if some aspects of the simulation did not go well. Keep the evaluation short, for example:

● Did you feel sufficiently prepared for the simulation (if no, what else would have helped you prepare?)
● What were the positive aspects of the simulation?
● What areas could be improved for future students?

A broader evaluation of effectiveness might include following up students in practice to assess knowledge, skills and behaviour.

Ultimately any resulting changes in practice within an organisation following the introduction of a simulation-based learning programme can be evaluated.

The process described above mirrors Kirkpatrick's (1996) four stage model for evaluating education and training moving from the specific individual experience of the student to the wider impact on the organisation and quality of service delivery.

STUDENTS' ATTITUDES TO SIMULATION

It is quite common for students to comment on how nervous they feel being observed, often telling you this before the simulation starts. Your ability to make a student feel at ease before, during and after a simulation exercise is crucial. On occasions you might need to step in and interrupt the simulation to help the student relax before continuing on, otherwise it may not achieve the learning planned.

It's not always possible, but you should try to prevent the students from attempting to blame any poor performance during a simulation exercise on an independent issue. If you have checked that every student feels able to attempt the exercise, both in terms of their understanding of what they are required to achieve, and that they feel well enough/relaxed enough to go ahead; then these issues should not be used as the basis of an excuse following the exercise. However, it is important that prior to the session commencing you should ask some simple and direct questions that will allow each student to declare confidentially the need for any reasonable adjustments they may require. For example, students with dyslexia may need more time to read any pre-session materials and any scenario provided to them.

GETTING SIMULATION RIGHT

While there is no guarantee that, despite a lot of planning and preparation, issues will not arise, good preparation will assist in troubleshooting the most common areas where simulation may not go as well as expected. Get this right and there is every chance that the simulation exercise will be an invaluable learning tool. Successful simulation can result in advanced preparation for practice learning opportunities as well as providing a student with alternative learning experiences while on practice placement.

So, remember a successful simulation relies upon:

- Ensuring everyone involved in the simulation has been prepared for their role and had staff development related to facilitating simulation.
- Ensuring that learning outcomes/expected student behaviours/time of simulation session are outlined ahead of the session.
- Agreeing and preparing the scenario/storyboard for simulation ahead of the session.
- Providing information sheets/packs in advance for 'patients or actors' that are participating in the simulation.
- Ensuring you have full equipment lists and are provided with 'set up' instructions.
- Allowing adequate time following the session for debriefing and feedback.

Action Points

1. Think about aspects of practice where simulation could be used in your clinical area.
2. Discuss possible scenarios you can use with colleagues and keep them in a folder ready to use when the opportunities arise.
3. Find out what resources are available in your organisation for simulated learning.
4. Arrange to attend simulation sessions at your own organisation or your local university.

Acknowledgment

Thank you to Sharon Elliott and Karen Murrell for contributing this chapter to the book.

RECOMMENDED READING

World Health Organisation: *Simulation in Nursing and Midwifery Nursing*, 2018, Available at: http://bit.ly/WHOSimulation.

Appendix 1

Facilitating a Simulation Session for a Subcutaneous Injection

LEARNING OUTCOMES

In this simulation session the student will be expected to:

- Demonstrate safe practice in relation to administering a subcutaneous injection
- Use communication skills to acknowledge the patient's feelings/concerns
- Provide the patient with accurate information regarding the subcutaneous injection
- Demonstrate professional behaviour throughout the procedure

Resources Required

- Sink area/alcohol hand rub
- Receiver/insulin needle
- Sterile water/labelled insulin
- Male simulated patient/actor sat in hospital bed with skin tone injection pad (with metal backing) strapped to abdomen
- Pyjamas
- Name band
- Medication chart
- Sharps bin
- Curtains/screen
- Gloves to be available

Chapter 13

Evaluating the Learning Experience

INTRODUCTION

It is a Nursing and Midwifery Council (NMC) requirement that programmes are evaluated and that this should be a partnership approach between both the university and practice learning partners. In addition, service users and key stakeholders should also be involved in the evaluation process (NMC, 2018e). It is important therefore to have an understanding of the different strategies available for evaluating the quality of the learning experience for students, including the role of practice supervisors and assessors and other health and social care professionals involved in supporting student learning. In addition to evaluating the student experience, every practice supervisor and practice assessor should take time to reflect on and evaluate their own performance and consider any professional development needs that may be required to enhance future performance in their role.

A Nurse's Survival Guide to Supervising and Assessing. https://doi.org/10.1016/B978-0-7020-8147-7.00013-2

WHY EVALUATION IS IMPORTANT

Just as it is important to evaluate the care you deliver to patients and clients, it is also important to evaluate the quality of a student's learning experience with you, not only to determine whether they had an effective learning experience themselves but also whether you were effective in your role as a practice supervisor or assessor. You might question whether you can have one without the other, but feedback from students suggests that whilst they can achieve their learning objectives and have their practice assessment document (PAD) completed, this does not necessarily mean that their experience was a positive one or that their practice supervisor or assessor has been supportive or effective in enabling them to fully access the range of learning opportunities available, or that they found the culture of the placement itself welcoming and supportive. However, where students have been well supported there is no question that their learning will have been enhanced. Evaluation therefore will provide you with an opportunity to consider improvements you can make in your role as a practice supervisor or assessor and in the wider learning environment that constitutes the placement and so enhance the learning experience for future students.

! Evaluation is essential to enable improvement of the learning environment for students and identify areas for your own personal development. Without evaluation you risk making the same mistakes over and over again.

WHEN TO EVALUATE

Evaluation is often seen as something that takes place at the end of a programme, but in fact evaluation is an ongoing process, you certainly wouldn't wait until the end of a patient's stay to evaluate whether your care had been effective, nor should you with a student! At university, educational staff will undertake a mid-module review to check that there are no problems with delivery or content so that any concerns can be responded to quickly and changes made where necessary. At the end of the module a more formal module evaluation will be undertaken and should hopefully not reveal any surprises. The university will also ask students to complete an evaluation of their placement on their return from practice. Whilst the results of these evaluations will be fed back to you there can be a time-lag hence the value of evaluations or review taking place whilst the student is on their placement.

Just as you give feedback at regular intervals to your student, it is also helpful to get feedback from them on the support you and other staff are providing them and whether their objectives and learning needs are being met. This should take place at regular intervals during a student's placement and gives the student an opportunity to raise any concerns which can be managed rather than waiting until the end when it is too late. Sometimes you may not be able to change what the student is unhappy about but the fact that you have asked and listened will go a long way with the student and it will have identified something that the placement can work on for the future. These quick reviews are an important part of a student placement but in addition a more formal evaluation at the end of each placement is valuable in enabling improvements for future students.

WHAT TO EVALUATE

Before deciding how you wish to evaluate the student experience you need to decide exactly what it is you wish to evaluate. Are you looking at the overall experience or do you want to focus on something specific? For example, you may have introduced something new such as an orientation booklet for students and want to focus on that, or you may have introduced new learning activities for students and want to know if they were valued by the students. Potential areas for evaluation are:

- the student's experience of the placement
- supporting students with additional needs
- the quality of the placement as a learning environment
- your own experience of supervising/assessing the student
- your role as a practice supervisor/assessor.

Each of these areas will overlap to a certain extent. A student's experience of their placement will be heavily influenced by the quality of the support they receive from you and the staff around you. Equally, a placement that is a poor environment for student learning is very likely to affect your ability to supervise and assess students effectively and so have an adverse impact on the quality of a student's learning experience with you.

THE STUDENT'S EXPERIENCE OF THEIR PLACEMENT

As discussed earlier, students are required by the university to evaluate their experience in practice and this contributes to the university quality assurance processes. Student evaluation is undertaken by the university and should be fed back to the placement providers at regular intervals. There is no standard evaluation tool, so each university will have a different approach to this and the type of questions they ask, although again some countries and regions have agreed on a single tool for their area to enable consistency in feedback to practice partners. If you have never seen the evaluations of your area completed by students placed with you, you should first check with your manager whether they have received them, and failing that contact the Link Lecturer attached to your area who should be able to provide you with copies or show you how to access them if they are available on line. The universities who place students with you will have agreed on an approach to make the evaluations available to each placement, so it is important that all staff in practice see these evaluations. The areas that the questions may cover are:

- preparation and orientation to the placement
- support from the practice supervisors and practice assessor
- learning opportunities and experience
- assessment process
- learning climate (what the area is like overall for learning)
- what improvements could be made.

The evaluation may use a Likert scale: for example, the student selects one of the following for each question: strongly agree, agree, neither agree or disagree, disagree, strongly disagree, or it could be a simple set of yes/no questions. These formats can be useful when large numbers of evaluations are collected as you can get a very quick sense check on areas of strength and areas for improvement. These types of (quantitative) evaluations may also offer the student the opportunity to make additional (qualitative) comments which can be useful in helping you to understand why they have given the scores they did. An alternative evaluation may focus far more on qualitative responses from the student, with a series of questions the student has to provide a written response to. Data from these take more time to collate but can be rich in information if the student takes the time to give a detailed response. They can also be less useful if the student gives very brief answers. An example of the type of questions that may be asked by a university regarding a student's experience of their placement can be found in Box 13.1.

BOX 13.1 Example of Some Questions From a Student Evaluation of Practice Placements

Question	Response
Were you orientated to the area within the first two days of placement?	Yes/No (delete as appropriate)
Please rate your experience of being supervised by Practice Supervisors in this placement (where 1 is not a good experience and 10 is an excellent experience)	1 2 3 4 5 6 7 8 9 10 (please ring)
Were you allocated a Practice Assessor within week one of your placement? If no, please comment.	Yes/No (delete as appropriate) Comment:
Please take this opportunity to identify a member of staff who has enhanced your practice placement experience and why?	Comment:

Developing Your Own Student Evaluation

You might like to consider a brief questionnaire/evaluation form that you give students at the end of their placement with you. The challenge with this approach is that because the student knows that you will be reading the answers they may not be as honest as they might be when they answer a questionnaire which is anonymous or completed once they are back at the university. To gain the most honest answers it is best to ask the student to complete the questionnaire after you have completed their practice assessment document and ask them to return it to you in a sealed envelope. The shorter the questionnaire the more likely it is that a student will complete it, so consider what you think are the important areas you want feedback on. You can use the feedback you receive to carry out a self-evaluation of the placement as a whole or to identify the aspects that that went well, and also the areas where changes need to be made to make it a better experience for future students. An example of some of the information you might like to receive feedback on could be:

- How did the orientation booklet help prepare you for your placement?
- How could we improve the orientation booklet?
- Did your orientation and induction to the placement take place on your first day?
- Did your initial interview take place in the first week of your placement?
- How many shifts did you undertake with your nominated practice supervisors during your placement?
- What went well on this placement?
- What areas could we do better in order to improve the learning experience for students?

You could also consider using a version of the Friends and Family Test (FTT) used widely by the NHS. For example:

- How likely are you to recommend this placement to friends and family if they needed care or treatment?
- How likely are you to recommend this placement to friends and family as a place to work?

Answers can range from the following:

- Extremely likely
- Likely
- Neither likely or unlikely
- Unlikely
- Extremely unlikely
- Don't know

An additional option after each of these two questions is to ask the student to give a reason or rationale for their answer.

Analysing Evaluations

Analysing student evaluations can be daunting and how you go about this will depend on how they are presented. Quantitative evaluations can be easier to analyse as it is primarily a case of counting up the scores. You can add up the scores for each question from a set of student evaluations and see which questions score well and those that score less well. Those that score less well may be areas that need to be acted on by you or your colleagues. You may need to determine what actions are needed.

Qualitative evaluations take more time to analyse, as the quality of the answers will depend on the quality of the questions, the student's understanding of the questions, and their ability to give an answer that is succinct and clear.

The more evaluations you can collect the more valuable they are. One single evaluation tells you what one particular student felt, whereas a number of evaluations allow you to see if there are any particular trends. Consider how you might respond to a comment by a student which says, '*I arrived on my first day, but no-one was expecting me, although they quickly allocated me a named practice supervisor*'. Consider why this may have occurred (you may wish to go back and look at Chapter 3) and what actions you would take to make sure it didn't happen again.

Possible reasons you may have given are:

- The nominated practice supervisor being off sick/on annual leave/on a different shift.
- An oversight by the manager of the placement.
- An error by the university in failing to inform the placement that a student was coming.

If only one student evaluation states this as an issue then this may have been a one-off occurrence; however, if more than one student highlights this as an issue then there is clearly a problem regarding either the way staff are allocated to students or the way that the university is informing the placement area when students will be coming to them. Both require actions which are easy to put in place. Possible strategies to ensure this won't happen are discussed in Chapter 3 and include:

- Ensuring that at least the nominated practice supervisor (and/or assessor) is on duty on a student's first day.
- Ensuring staff who are allocated a student are not due to take leave at the start of a student's placement with them.
- Identifying a specific person to be responsible for allocation of practice supervisors/assessors to students.
- Discussing with the university how allocations are communicated.

Whilst the majority of students are very positive about their practice supervisors and assessors and their placement experience there will be some students who will be less than happy with their experience. If you receive less than positive evaluations, it is important to consider why this may be.

> ! If a student evaluates your practice area as poor in any given area, then try to account for why this might be. Don't be defensive; look for specific objective evidence to support the student evaluation and consider why they may have felt that way.

Poorly Written Evaluations

Evaluations have no value unless there are actions that arise out of them. If all answers are positive then it can be more difficult to develop an action plan, but it is also worth considering whether the evaluation form is asking the right questions or if they are leading questions so pushing students to make a specific response. A question like 'How can we improve the induction booklet?' implies the booklet needs improving. Equally all closed questions which force a 'Yes' or 'No' answer without asking the student to give a reason for their answer leave you with no idea why they answered yes or no, so rating scales or asking students to explain why they have given a yes or no answer is far more likely to provide information that can help you. If you find your evaluations do not give you information that can guide you on areas to improve, then consider talking to a practice educator in your organisation or your Link Lecturer for advice. Equally a quick search on the internet can provide you with examples used by placement providers and universities that you could use as a starting point.

EVALUATING THE QUALITY OF THE PLACEMENT AS A LEARNING ENVIRONMENT

As well as considering student feedback on their experience, you may wish to consider other feedback about your practice area as a learning environment to help you identify areas for improvement. The most common tool that is specifically focussed on the placement as a learning environment is the educational audit.

Educational Audits

Universities are required by the NMC to *regularly review all learning environments and provide assurance that they are safe and effective* (NMC, 2018e, p. 8). This traditionally takes the form of an educational audit of each learning environment in the practice area where students are placed. The rationale for this is to ensure that the placement:

- Has sufficient resources to support the number of students who will be placed there at any one time
- Has staff who are acting as practice supervisors or practice assessors who meet the NMC's SSSA standards (2018b) and have been suitably prepared for their role
- Provides the appropriate learning opportunities to enable the students to meet programme learning outcomes (i.e. your placement may be appropriate for students at any point on a programme or only appropriate for a specific part of a programme)
- Provides opportunities for learning with and from other health and social care professionals
- Has nurses, midwives and nursing associates (as appropriate) who understand and comply with the NMC's *Code* (2018b) in supporting student learning in practice
- Meets key health and safety regulations
- Has key policies in place relevant to student learning (e.g. raising concerns)

The audits are usually undertaken in partnership with the staff in the placement and will take place at regularly agreed intervals. Both the university and the placement will retain a copy of the completed audit so you should be able to get a copy of your most recent audit very easily – or it may be available online. The audit also enables the university and practice to identify specific areas in a placement that need further development to assure the quality of the learning environment for students as well as for identifying areas of good practice that can be disseminated to other placement areas. The most common actions tend to be around preparation of staff to become practice supervisors or assessors in order that there are sufficient to support the number of students allocated to the area. If there are action plans in the audit it is essential that these are responded to and reviewed to ensure completion. An action plan without any actions taking place has no value!

! Ask to look at the education audit for your practice area. It will typically be held by the manager and will highlight any particular areas for improvement.

Local and National Audits

Other reports which might inform you about the quality of your area and therefore potentially indicate its quality as a learning environment are:

- internal audits, for example numbers of pressure sores, medication errors, staffing levels, infection rates
- friends and family surveys

- patient surveys
- staff surveys
- Care Quality Commission (CQC) reports.

Although the CQC reports look at an organisation as a whole, they can also pick up on both good practice and areas of concern for specific wards/departments. Both the NMC and universities monitor CQC reports as they are indicators of potential concerns regarding the quality of placement areas as learning environments. Where a CQC visit results in serious concerns the NMC will contact all universities that place students with that placement provider to ask what actions the university has taken to mitigate any impact on the quality of student learning. This may be a reduction in student numbers or closure to specific placement areas to students to give the areas an opportunity to make improvements before taking students again.

EVALUATING YOUR OWN EXPERIENCE OF SUPPORTING STUDENTS

There are a number of different strategies that you can use to evaluate your own experience of supporting students and your effectiveness as a practice supervisor or assessor. It also an expectation of the NMC that you reflect on your role (NMC, 2019b) and uphold the standards set out in the *Code* (NMC, 2018a), specifically:

9.2 gather and reflect on feedback from a variety of sources, using it to improve your practice and performance

9.4 support students' and colleagues' learning to help them develop their professional competence and confidence

20.8 act as a role model of professional behaviour for students and newly qualified nurses, midwives and nursing associates to aspire to.

This section will look at four different methods that you can use to either self-evaluate your own experience or gain feedback from others about your performance as a practice supervisor or assessor.

Strengths, Weaknesses, Opportunities and Threats Analysis

SWOT stands for **S**trengths, **W**eaknesses, **O**pportunities and **T**hreats. It is a quick and easy tool that can be used to examine both your own performance and the practice area in which you work as a learning environment for students.

! Look at Box 13.2 and undertake a SWOT analysis using the headings and questions.

Reflection

All students are required to reflect on their practice, and it is an NMC professional requirement of you as a registered nurse that you too reflect on your practice as part of your revalidation every 3 years (NMC, 2019a). So, reflecting on your role as a practice supervisor or practice assessor is not only good practice but also valuable preparation for your revalidation every 3 years. If you undertake them after each student you have supported has completed their placement with you, then you will have a wealth of examples ready for use at your revalidation meeting with your confirmer. In addition, they can also be used as part of your annual appraisal. Undertaking regular reflections also allows you to become familiar with the reflective models that students use and also to appreciate how challenging this can be at times but also how valuable. There are a range of reflective models or frameworks that you can use, and it is worth trying several to see which one suits you best. If you are unfamiliar with them then it is probably a good idea to talk to the students you have allocated to your area or the Link Lecturer from their university to find out what models they use. Models can be circular in format (see Fig 12.1 in Chapter 12) or a list of questions that you answer, but all have common elements:

- Looking back on what happened.
- Examining thoughts and feelings about what happened.
- Identifying what went well and not so well and why.
- Identifying what you have learnt from the experience.
- Considering how you will respond to a similar situation in the future, changes you need to make or actions you need to undertake to improve future practice.

When reflecting you can choose a specific element of the supervisor/assessor relationship (e.g. giving feedback), a particular moment that went well or not so well (e.g. demonstrating a skill) or look at the whole period of supporting a student. It is useful to record your reflections in a journal (handwritten or on a

---

BOX 13.2 Strengths, Weaknesses, Opportunities and Threats Analysis

SWOT Analysis

Think about students you have supported/supervised/assessed over the last year and write a few notes under each of the headings listed below:

Strengths	Weaknesses
What were the strong points of your support to students? What is the evidence?	What areas could you improve upon? Why do you think this?
Opportunities	Threats
What opportunities are there to enable you to improve as a practice supervisor or assessor?	What are the threats to you in acting as supervisor or assessor? What prevents you supporting students as well as you would like?

computer). This allows you to look back over time to see what you have learnt and how you have developed. It is also a good way of picking up on common themes. For example, you may find that you have similar problems with each student such as giving feedback, and this can focus your attention on an area in which you need to develop specific skills. Box 13.3 offers a series of questions that can help you to reflect on a recent experience supervising/assessing a student.

Guided Reflection

Reflective practice can be a solitary exercise and requires you to have a high degree of self-awareness and the ability to be critically honest about your actions and feelings. Sharing your reflections with another person can be helpful as another person can challenge your actions, feelings and assumptions and so help you to become more aware of your thoughts and behaviours. If clinical supervision is available in your workplace then make use of this, or ask a more experienced member of staff if they would be willing to provide clinical supervision for your role as a practice supervisor or assessor.

! Try to discuss the experiences of everyone when you have had groups of students with colleagues regularly at team meetings. Issues can be highlighted, and problems resolved very quickly if they are talked about openly and constructively.

Evaluating the Experience of Practice Supervisors and Assessors in Supporting Students

An alternative approach to evaluating student placements is to evaluate the experience of the practice supervisors and assessors who support students on a placement (or within your organisation). This can be a valuable way of identifying a number of core factors that could impact the experience of both the supervisors and assessors and therefore potentially on the student's own experience of their placement. It can enable you to get a sense of their understanding

---

BOX 13.3 A Checklist for Personal Reflection

Think back to a student for whom you have recently acted as a practice supervisor or assessor, and answer the following questions about your experience with that student:

1. How did you feel about the relationship between yourself and your student? What was good about it? What did you feel uncomfortable about? Why?
2. What went well during their placement with you? Why do you think this was?
3. What did not go well? Why do you think this was?
4. What could you have done to have improved the situation?
5. What have you learnt about yourself as a practice supervisor or practice assessor from supporting this student?
6. How will you use this new knowledge to improve your skills for the future?

of their role, how well prepared they feel and whether they know what to do in different situations. Box 13.4 provides some questions you might want to consider. If a member of staff says 'No' to any questions then this can indicate areas for their development.

LEARNING FROM EVALUATIONS, AUDITS AND SURVEYS

No-one likes to hear bad news and it is important not to take evaluations that are critical of you or the placement where you work too personally. Rather, consider what may have caused the student to be critical and whether they have justification for their comments. Reflect on whether there were any difficulties with particular students or in the placement itself at the time that they were with you that may have led them to evaluate their experience negatively. Examples of factors that may lead to negative evaluations are:

● Staff shortages impacting on the level of support and supervision offered to a student.
● Changes in service delivery (e.g. ward closure or moves or changing its specialty).
● Lack of understanding by practice supervisors/assessors about the student's programme/learning outcomes/needs/practice assessment document.
● Student failed by practice assessor.

BOX 13.4 A Check List to Evaluate the Understanding and Confidence of Practice Supervisors or Practice Assessors in Supporting Students

1. I am a Practice Supervisor/a Practice Assessor (delete role that does not apply).
2. I have completed a programme/workshop to prepare me for my role.
3. I feel confident in my role as a practice supervisor/practice assessor.
4. I know where to access resources to support student learning on placement.
5. I understand the actions I need to take if problems arise with a student's behaviour.
6. I have received information/guidance on how to manage a failing student.
7. I have had opportunities to discuss the management of the failing student (formally or informally).
8. I have been offered opportunities to participate in the recruitment & selection of student nurses at my local university.
9. I am aware of the Disability Discrimination Act and how it relates to me as an NHS employee and in supporting students.
10. I know who the link teachers are for my practice area.
11. I know how to access help if I am experiencing difficulties in my role as a practice supervisor or assessor.
12. I know whom to contact at the university if I have a query or need help with a student.

The first two points should have been anticipated by the manager and actions taken in advance of students coming to the placement. Any changes to a placement or reductions in staffing levels should be communicated to the university in order that they can reconsider whether students should be allocated to you or whether students at a different stage of their programme are more suited. The third point is a failing by the practice assessor/supervisor to fulfil their responsibility to ensure that they are up to date with the students' programme and practice assessment process, but this can be easily rectified by contacting the Link Lecturer to your areas to ask for an update for staff. The last point cannot be so easily anticipated but it is important to consider when a student has been failed and evaluates a placement negatively, whether they were supported appropriately during their placement and whether the assessment process was fair and just.

The feedback you receive from students will provide invaluable insight into your own performance. It can also be a valuable way to find out how your approach to supervision or assessment is perceived by students. You may like to use your self-reflective checklist and the feedback from students to answer the following questions.

1. What aspects of student support, supervision or assessment do you excel in?
2. How can you share these aspects with others and encourage them to do likewise?
3. In what areas do you not achieve well, or receive poor feedback on?
4. What can you do to strengthen your weaker areas?
5. Based on your last experience with a student, what will you definitely repeat with future students?
6. Based on your last experience with a student, what will you do differently?

! Share good practice with others in your team so that you can learn from each other.

ENHANCING THE LEARNING ENVIRONMENT

Discussions with students about their practice experience when they return to the university reveal common threads on what has made a positive learning experience for them. The most important is the relationship developed with the practice supervisor and practice assessor. Students describe a positive relationship as welcoming, supportive, willing, friendly and approachable. Other factors that students report back that have made a good placement for them are:

● The student was expected and welcomed.
● Information was available on how to prepare for the placement.
● The staff were interested in the student and the student felt part of the team.

- The nominated practice supervisor was able to work regularly with the student.
- The student was given opportunities to learn new skills.
- The staff were seen as knowledgeable.

There are a number of activities that you could consider undertaking to make your area a positive learning environment for students, most of which, once done, only need a small amount of time to maintain. Examples of such activities include:

- Sending out pre-placement emails and/or induction/orientation booklets to students to welcome them to the area.
- Ensuring your orientation pack is up to date and includes information relevant to the range of students placed with you.
- Providing a student noticeboard with contact details and learning opportunities.
- An easily accessible resource folder (or site on the organisation's intranet) for practice supervisors/assessors and students.

LEARNING FROM FEEDBACK

The best outcome from a practice placement is that both you and your student have had a positive, rewarding experience. Not only will you have had an opportunity for facilitating learning experiences, you will have made a valuable contribution to a student's journey towards registration. If experiences during the practice placement are less than satisfactory then it is important that you view these as opportunities to learn and improve, rather than seeing them as negatives and losing motivation. Seek feedback about your skills in supporting student learning from a wide variety of students and use this information to improve your own skills in supporting and developing students. In this way you are compliant with the NMC *Code* requirement that you *keep your knowledge and skills up to date, taking part in appropriate and regular learning and professional development activities that aim to maintain and develop your competence and improve your performance* (NMC, 2018a, Standard 22.3).

Action Points

1. Ask to see the student evaluations about your placement twice a year so you can identify what is working well and what needs improving.
2. Keep a reflective journal that records both the positive experiences and the challenges you have experienced with students and any student feedback you receive; you can then use this at your NMC Revalidation meeting with your manager.
3. Set up a forum on your workplace to share good practice with others.
4. Participate in the next educational audit of your workplace.

Appendix 1

Extract of Skills from The NMC Standards of Proficiency for Registered Nurses (NMC, 2018d)

Annexe A: Communication and relationship skills

3. Evidence-based, best practice communication skills and approaches for providing therapeutic interventions
   - **3.1** motivational interview techniques
   - **3.2** solution focused therapies
   - **3.3** reminiscence therapies
   - **3.4** talking therapies
   - **3.5** de-escalation strategies and techniques
   - **3.6** cognitive behavioural therapy techniques
   - **3.7** play therapy
   - **3.8** distraction and diversion strategies
   - **3.9** positive behaviour support approaches

Annexe B: Nursing procedures

Part 1: Procedures for assessing people's needs for person-centred care

1. Use evidence-based, best practice approaches to take a history, observe, recognise and accurately assess people of all ages:
   - **1.1** mental health and wellbeing status
     - **1.1.1** signs of mental and emotional distress or vulnerability
     - **1.1.2** cognitive health status and wellbeing
     - **1.1.3** signs of cognitive distress and impairment
     - **1.1.4** behavioural distress based needs

1.1.5 signs of mental and emotional distress including agitation, aggression and challenging behaviour

1.1.6 signs of self-harm and/or suicidal ideation

1.2 physical health and wellbeing

1.2.1 symptoms and signs of physical ill health

1.2.2 symptoms and signs of physical distress

1.2.3 symptoms and signs of deterioration and sepsis.

2. Use evidence-based, best practice approaches to undertake the following procedures:

2.1 take, record and interpret vital signs manually and via technological devices

2.2 undertake venepuncture and cannulation and blood sampling, interpreting normal and common abnormal blood profiles and venous blood gases

2.3 set up and manage routine electrocardiogram (ECG) investigations and interpret normal and commonly encountered abnormal traces

2.4 manage and monitor blood component transfusions

2.5 manage and interpret cardiac monitors, infusion pumps, blood glucose monitors and other monitoring devices

2.6 accurately measure weight and height, calculate body mass index and recognise healthy ranges and clinically significant low/high readings

2.7 undertake a whole body systems assessment including respiratory, circulatory, neurological, musculoskeletal, cardiovascular and skin status

2.8 undertake chest auscultation and interpret findings

2.9 collect and observe sputum, urine, stool and vomit specimens, undertaking routine analysis and interpreting findings

2.10 measure and interpret blood glucose levels

2.11 recognise and respond to signs of all forms of abuse

2.12 undertake, respond to and interpret neurological observations and assessments

2.13 identify and respond to signs of deterioration and sepsis

2.14 administer basic mental health first aid

2.15 administer basic physical first aid

2.16 recognise and manage seizures, choking and anaphylaxis, providing appropriate basic life support

2.17 recognise and respond to challenging behaviour, providing appropriate safe holding and restraint.

References

Adamson E, King L, Foy L, et al. Feedback in clinical practice: enhancing the students' experience through action research. *Nurse Educ Pract*. 2018;31:48–53.

All Wales practice assessment document and ongoing record of achievement; 2020. Available at: https://heiw.nhs.wales/programmes/once-for-wales-2020/.

Anderson LW, Krathwohl DR, Airasian PW, et al. *A Taxonomy for Learning, Teaching, and Assessing: A Revision of Bloom's Taxonomy of Educational Objectives*. 1st ed. New York, NY: Longman; 2001.

Bazian Ltd. *RCN Mentorship Project 2015: From Today's Support in Practice to Tomorrow's Vision for Excellence*. London: RCN; 2016.

Bloom BS, Engelhart MD, Furst EJ, Hill WH, Krathwohl DR. *Taxonomy of Educational Objectives: The Classification of Educational Goals. Handbook 1: Cognitive Domain*. New York, NY: David McKay; 1956.

Brown P, Jones A, Davies J. Shall I tell my mentor? Exploring the mentor-student relationship and its impact on students' raising concerns on clinical placement. *J Clin Nurs*. 2020;29:3298–3310.

Burke H, Mancuso L. Social cognitive theory, metacognition, and simulation learning in nursing education. *J Nurs Educ*. 2012;51(10):543–548.

Calleja P, Harvey T, Fox A, Carmichael M. Feedback and clinical practice improvement: a tool to assist workplace supervisors and students. *Nurse Educ Pract*. 2016;17:167–173.

Cant R, Cooper S, Sussex R, Bogossian F. What's in a name? clarifying the nomenclature of virtual simulation. *Clin Simul Nurs*. 2019;27:26–30.

Dave RH. Psychomotor levels. In: Armstrong RJ, ed. *Developing and Writing Behavioural Objectives*. Tucson: Educational Innovators Press; 1970.

Directive 2005/36/EC Directive 2005/36/EC of the European Parliament and of the Council of 7 September 2005 on the recognition of professional qualifications. *Off J Eur Union*. 2005;L 255:22–142. Available at: http://eurlex.europa.eu/LexUriServ/LexUriServ.do?uri=OJ:L:2005: 255:0022:0142:EN:PDF.

Donaldson I, Stainer L, Cooper K. Introducing an online portfolio for practice placement assessments. *Nurs Times*. 2020;116(2):53–56.

Duffy K. *Failing Students: A Qualitative Study of Factors that Influence the Decisions Regarding Assessment of Students' Competence in Practice*. Glasgow, Scotland: Glasgow Caledonian University; 2003.

Duffy K, Hardicre J. Supporting failing students in practice 2: management. *Nurs Times*. 2007;103(48):28–29.

Duffy K. Providing constructive feedback to students during mentoring. *Nurs Stand*. 2013;27(31):50–56.

Elcock K. *How to Succeed on Nursing Placements*. London: Learning Matters; 2020.

Felton A, Wright N. Simulation in mental health nurse education: the development, implementation and evaluation of an educational innovation. *Nurse Educ Pract*. 2017;26:46–52.

Francis R. *Report of the Mid Staffordshire NHS Foundation Trust Public Inquiry Executive Summary*. London: The Stationery Office; 2013.

Francis R. Freedom to speak up; 2015. Available at: http://freedomtospeakup.org.uk/the-report/.

Fulton J. The archaeology and genealogy of mentorship in English nursing. *Nurs Inq*. 2015;22:39–49.

Gamble AS. Simulation in undergraduate paediatric nursing curriculum: evaluation of a complex 'ward for a day' education program. *Nurse Educ Pract*. 2017;23:40–47.

Gibbs G. *Learning by Doing: A Guide to Teaching and Learning Methods*. Oxford: Further Education Unit, Oxford Polytechnic; 1988.

Harder BN. Use of simulation in teaching and learning in health sciences: a systematic review. *J Nurs Educ*. 2010;49(1):23–28.

Health Education England. Research evidence of the impact of generational differences on the NHS workforce; 2019. Available at: https://allcatsrgrey.org.uk/wp/download/management/human_resources/Generational-Differences-Deep-Dive.pdf.

HESA. What do HE students study? Personal characteristics; 2019. Available at: https://www.hesa.ac.uk/data-and-analysis/students/what-study/characteristics.

Hill R, Woodward M, Arthur A. Collaborative Learning in Practice (CLIP): evaluation of a new approach to clinical learning. *Nurse Educ Today*. 2020;85:104295.

Hirdle J, Keeley S, Bareham S, Allan L. A collaborative learning model for student nurses in child mental health. *Nurs Times*. 2020;116(1):50–52.

Honey P, Mumford A. *The Learning Styles Questionnaire, 80-Item Version*. Maidenhead, UK: Peter Honey Publications; 2006.

Hunt LA, McGee P, Gutteridge R, Hughes M. Assessment of student nurses in practice: a comparison of theoretical and practical assessment results in England. *Nurs Educ Today*. 2012;32:351–355.

Hunt LA, McGee P, Gutteridge R, Hughes M. Manipulating mentors' assessment decisions: do underperforming student nurses use coercive strategies to influence mentors' practical assessment decisions? *Nurse Educ Pract*. 2016;20:154–162.

IFF Research. *Evaluation of the NMC Pre-registration Standards: Summary Report*. London: NMC; 2015.

Jaye P, Thomas L, Reedy G. 'The Diamond': a structure for simulation debrief. *Clin Teach*. 2015;12(3):171–175.

Jones K, Warren A, Davies A. *Mind the Gap. Summary Report from Birmingham and Solihull Local Education and Training Council Every Student Counts Project*; 2015. Available at: https://www.nhsemployers.org/-/media/Employers/Documents/Plan/Mind-the-Gap-Smaller.pdf.

Kirkpatrick DL. Evaluation. In: Craig RL, Bittel LR, eds. *Training & Development Handbook. American Society for Training and Development*. New York, NY: McGraw-Hill Book Co; 1996.

Kolbe M, Grande B, Spahn D. Briefing and debriefing during simulation-based training and beyond: content, structure, attitude and setting. *Best Pract Res Clin Anaesthesiol*. 2015;29:87–96.

Lovegrove MJ. *RePAIR: Reducing Pre-registration Attrition and Improving Retention Report*. London: Health Education England; 2018.

MacDonald K, Paterson K, Wallar J. Nursing students' experience of practice placements. *Nurs Stand*. 2016;31(10):44–50.

Major R, Tetley J. Effects of dyslexia on registered nurses in practice. *Nurse Educ Pract*. 2019;35:7–13.

Morley D, Wilson K, Holbery N. *Facilitating Learning in Practice. A Research-Based Approach to Challenges and Solutions*. Abingdon: Routledge; 2019.

NHS Education for Scotland. A National Framework for Practice Supervisors, Practice Assessors and Academic Assessors in Scotland; 2019. Available at: www.nes.scot.nhs.uk/media/4354527/scottish_approach_to_student_supervision_and_assessment_interactive.pdf.

North H, Kennedy M, Wray J. Are mentors failing to fail underperforming student nurses? An integrative literature review. *Br J Nurs*. 2019;28(4):250–255.

Nursing and Midwifery Council. *Standards for Learning and Assessment in Practice*. London: NMC; 2008.

Nursing and Midwifery Council. *General Medical Council. Openness and Honesty When Things Go Wrong: The Professional Duty of Candour*. London: NMC; 2015.

Nursing and Midwifery Council. *The Code: Professional Standards of Practice and Behaviour for Nurses, Midwives and Nursing Associates*. London: NMC; 2018a.

Nursing and Midwifery Council. *Realising Professionalism: Standards for Education and Training Part 2: Standards for Student Supervision and Assessment*. London: NMC; 2018b.

Nursing and Midwifery Council. *Realising Professionalism: Standards for Education and Training Part 3: Standards for Pre-registration Nursing Programmes*. London: NMC; 2018c.

Nursing and Midwifery Council. *Future Nurse: Standards of Proficiency for Registered Nurses*. London: NMC; 2018d.

Nursing and Midwifery Council. *Realising Professionalism: Standards for Education and Training Part 1: Standards Framework for Nursing and Midwifery Education*. London: NMC; 2018e.

Nursing and Midwifery Council. *Supporting Information on Standards for Student Supervision and Assessment*. London: NMC; 2018f.

Nursing and Midwifery Council. *Revalidation*. London: NMC; 2019a.

Nursing and Midwifery Council. *Guidance on Health and Character*. London: NMC; 2019b.

Nursing and Midwifery Council. London: NMC; We regulate nursing associates. Available at: https://www.nmc.org.uk/about-us/our-role/who-we-regulate/nursing-associates/ 2020.

Once for Wales. Student evaluation of practice learning experiences; 2020. Available at: https://heiw.nhs.wales/programmes/once-for-wales-2020/.

Ossenberg C, Henderson A, Mitchell M. What attributes guide best practice for effective feedback? A scoping review. *Adv Health Sci Educ*. 2019;24:383–401.

Pan London Practice Learning Group. Pan London Practice Assessment Document; 2019a. Available at: https://plplg.uk/plpad-2-0/.

Pegasus. Generation Z: the future of health and wellbeing, behavioural differences between generations; 2018. Available at: http://thisispegasus.co.uk/content/themes/pegasus/build/images/genz.pdf.

Pendleton D, Schofield T, Tate P, Havelock P. *The Consultation: An Approach to Learning and Teaching*. Oxford: University Press Oxford; 1984.

Reynolds L, Attenborough J, Halse J. Nurses as educators: creating teachable moments in practice. *Nurs Times*. 2020;116(2):25–28.

Royal College of Nursing. *BREXIT: Royal College of Nursing Priorities Overview*. London: RCN; 2019.

Royal Pharmaceutical Society. A competency framework for all prescribers; 2016. Available from: https://www.rpharms.com/resources/frameworks/prescribers-competency-framework.

Rudolph JW, Simon R, Dufresne RL, Raemer DB. There's no such thing as "nonjudgmental" debriefing: a theory and method for debriefing with good judgment. *Simul Healthc*. 2006;1(1):49–55.

Saunder L, Knight R-A. CitySCaPE: moving beyond indifference in education for pre-registration nurses about learning disability. *Nurse Educ Pract*. 2017;26:82–88.

Tremayne P, Hunt L. Has anyone seen the student? Creating a welcoming practice environment for students. *Br J Nurs*. 2019;28(6):369–373.

UCAS. Nursing by individual age. UCAS Undergraduate Sector-Level End of Cycle Data Resources; 2019. Available at: https://www.ucas.com/data-and-analysis.

Williamson G, Bunce J, Kane A, Jamison C, Clarke D. Investigating the implementation of a collaborative learning in practice model of nurse education in a community placement cluster: a qualitative study. *Open Learn J*. 2020;14:39–48.

Willis P. *Quality With Compassion: The Future of Nursing Education. Report of the Willis Commission.* London: RCN; 2012.

Willis P. *Raising the Bar. Shape of Caring: A Review of the Future Education and Training of Registered Nurses and Care Assistants.* London: Health Education England/NMC; 2015.

World Health Organization. *Towards a Common Language for Functioning, Disability and Health: ICF The International Classification of Functioning, Disability and Health.* Geneva: WHO; 2002.

Wyllie E, Batley B. Skills for safe practice – a qualitative study to evaluate the use of simulation in safeguarding children teaching for pre-registration children's nurses. *Nurse Educ Pract.* 2019;34:85–89.

Zigmont JJ, Kappus LJ, Sudikoff SN. The 3D model of debriefing: defusing, discovering, and deepening. *Semin Perinatol.* 2011;35(2):52–58.

Index

Note: Page numbers followed by *b* indicate boxes, *f* indicate figures and *t* indicate tables.